T0095679

How to
LIVE LONG
and
LIKE IT

The Longevity Diet

By Jim Heckathorn

WESTBOW®
PRESS
A DIVISION OF THOMAS NELSON
& ZONDERVAN

Copyright © 2015 Jim Heckathorn.

All rights reserved. No part of this book may be used or reproduced by any means, graphic, electronic, or mechanical, including photocopying, recording, taping or by any information storage retrieval system without the written permission of the publisher except in the case of brief quotations embodied in critical articles and reviews.

WestBow Press books may be ordered through booksellers or by contacting:

WestBow Press
A Division of Thomas Nelson & Zondervan
1663 Liberty Drive
Bloomington, IN 47403
www.westbowpress.com
1 (866) 928-1240

Because of the dynamic nature of the Internet, any web addresses or links contained in this book may have changed since publication and may no longer be valid. The views expressed in this work are solely those of the author and do not necessarily reflect the views of the publisher, and the publisher hereby disclaims any responsibility for them.

Any people depicted in stock imagery provided by Thinkstock are models, and such images are being used for illustrative purposes only. Certain stock imagery © Thinkstock.

Unless otherwise noted, all scripture quotations are taken from the New King James Version. Copyright © 1979, 1980, 1982 by Thomas Nelson, Inc. Used by permission. All rights reserved.

ISBN: 978-1-4908-6341-2 (sc)
ISBN: 978-1-4908-6342-9 (hc)
ISBN: 978-1-4908-6340-5 (e)

Library of Congress Control Number: 2014922160

Printed in the United States of America.

WestBow Press rev. date: 1/5/2015

Contents

Foreword

The practice of medicine has typically concentrated upon the physical, mental and emotional aspects of healing. I find that addressing spiritual disease is beneficial for all who are willing. Hope is so much more evident with Jesus in the center of any situation. He is wonderfully faithful and always answers our prayers even though they may not be answered how we thought they should be answered.

Many of my patients received answers and solutions after being helped to identify what the real issues are and then praying for help. I quite humbly say that I put the bandage on but the Lord is the one who does the true healing.

Diet and exercise are mainstays of the recommendations I give my patients. There is a plethora of information available in bookstores and on line, as well as at specialty stores. The question becomes whom do you believe? Supplements that were thought to be safe a decade ago are now known to have potential adverse effects. Just where is the truth?

Some years ago we experienced a supernatural miracle during a surgical procedure at our small clinic. The event rocked my world that day and when I woke the next morning still reeling over it's significance, I had knowledge of a truth that resonated in my core and today resonates even more. I "knew that I knew that I knew" that every word in the Bible was true. I didn't know how or have any of the specifics, but I knew that it was true. For someone who had never even read the entire Bible from cover to cover, I thought it was an odd conclusion to the previous day's event. This sparked an interest in searching for the truth and a journey that is continuing to unfold daily.

I have wondered for some time what the Bible says about how to nourish the human body that God created. How do I know that He created our bodies? I probably have to say common sense and years studying science. From biochemistry, microbiology and molecular biology to astronomy and the heavens, they all scream the same thing: complexity!

Just study how our genetic material is copied and passed on from cell to cell, how the blood clots after an injury, or how we are able to fight infections.

The human body is so detailed and complex. Even attaching a flagellum of a unicellular bacterium has a complex and ordered special assembly. I've not understood how this was to happen by chance. Apparently mathematicians have tried to calculate the chance of something like this occurring spontaneously. It's really impossible to consider rationally that biological life, as we know it, happened randomly.

Looking to biblical references I was perplexed in the past about how John the Baptist ate wild locusts out in the wilderness. "John's clothes were woven from coarse camel hair, and he wore a leather belt around his waist. For food he ate locusts and wild honey." (Matthew 3:4 NLT) He played such a key role but munching on grasshoppers was something that made me cringe. What a relief to find out that the locust is a type of fruit found in the Middle East. He may have had insects available periodically, but they were not abundant enough to supply a person's dietary needs. The website www.antipas.net gives us the following information: "Leguminous evergreen tree (Ceratonia siliqua) native to the East Mediterranean region and cultivated elsewhere. It is sometimes known as locust, or Saint John's Bread', in the belief that the 'locusts' on which John the Baptist fed were carob pods. The tree, about 50 ft (15 m) tall, bears compound, glossy leaves with thick leaflets. Its red flowers are followed by flat, leathery pods that contain 5-15 hard brown seeds embedded in a sweet, edible pulp that tastes similar to chocolate." Eating honey and chocolate sounds much more appealing.

Whether from a perspective of common sense or divine design, it makes sense to see what nutritional guidance comes from the Bible.

I welcome Reverend Jim Heckathorn's fresh approach at looking at this timely issue

Dr. Vicke Wooll, MD., MPH

Authors Note: In a personal conversation with Dr. Wooll, she agreed that longevity is not all in the genes an individual inherits. She emphasized the importance of the healthy integrity of the cellular structure of the body for health and longevity. The information in this book is intended to inform individuals about what they can do to maintain this healthy cellular structure. Dr. Wooll heartily agrees that individuals must be primarily responsible for their own healthcare. Good health results from informing yourself of the things you can do daily to maintain your good health. To this end the information found herein will be invaluable.

Dr. Vicki Wooll MD., MPH (Master of Public Health) maintains her family practice in medicine as proprietor of Eagle Creek Family Medicine in Eagle, Idaho. She received her degrees at the University of California, Los Angeles, and the Central University of Venezuela, and she completed the Corpus Cristi Family Practice residency program. Upon completing residency, she was awarded the Henry F. Harren, MD. Award of Excellence in Family Practice and received certification from the American Board of Family Medicine. Dr. Wooll practices holistic medicine in which she treats the whole person through focused individual care. She enjoys her involvement with her family and in community nonprofit organizations and medical mission work that has included multiple trips to Africa, India, and Central and South America.

Introduction

You are holding in your hands a complete book on anti-aging skills that will enlighten you concerning the human body and its requirements for weight management, wellness and other areas of concern necessary to living long and living well. It is actually possible for you to slow the clock or even reverse the signs of aging in your body. As you read you may be surprised to learn what it takes to live a good long life. One thing for sure is that you can't leave it to chance.

This book provides some little known knowledge that will help you to learn and apply the ten steps that will greatly enhance your opportunity to live long and like it. Actually, in many respects, this book is a survival guide, especially regarding your physical and mental well-being and your ability to sustain yourself financially through a lengthy retirement. Life is never easy, but the information in this book will make it easier.

Every living person wants a happy, healthy meaningful life wherein he or she can experience the joy of living. When the Creator put man and woman upon the earth, He intended that their existence would be long and deeply satisfying. The author wants you to know that you are able to achieve this goal.

One of the best features that you will gain from this book is how you can achieve your optimal body mass (weight for height). Can you imagine how much better you will look and feel when you have shed your few extra pounds and reduced the size of your waist?

The Longevity Diet is the result of the work of many researchers who have scoured the world's cultures known to demonstrate longevity, and of the scientific researchers continually seeking to discover the factors that contribute to living long and living well. The Longevity Diet is not a fad diet nor merely a compilation of foods to eat, or to avoid, but it is a lifestyle to be learned and lived to improve quality of life. The researchers have formulated those factors which have been applied experientially to prove the things that have been learned. In the Longevity Diet, the best known dietary research has been brought together for the benefit of longevity-minded men and women. Those who have the desire to live long and live well and who will commit to studying and diligently applying the diet plan can be assured of a measure of success regardless of the stage of life they are in. The earlier in life these things are learned and applied, the better, but even senior citizens can derive positive benefits by adopting this lifestyle.

Preface
A Philosophy of Life

The will to live is innate in the soul of man as in all living creatures. Longevity of life is most highly valued when life is viewed as more than just staying alive as long as possible. The pinnacle of life is to breathe fresh air, see the sunlight, and know that your life is a part of something greater than life itself. Life is valued when each new day is viewed as an opportunity to explore the wonders of life, the richness of life, and the deep meaning of life; to reach for something higher than yourself and to make your contribution to the grand scheme of which you are a part.

The years with which you are blessed are valued when your life is lived deliberately and actively in a manner that gives purpose and meaning to life; lifting your inner being each day to greater heights which culminate in your ultimate fulfillment. Life is more than satisfying your needs and desires; it is the striving toward your greatest possibilities to make your most profound contribution to humanity. However great or small your contribution may be, it will uplift your soul and inspire those who are aware of you and will look up to you.

Above all else, life is most uniquely valued when you realize that all life is created by and endowed with love by our creator. To perceive that love and to be fully enveloped in it is the ultimate pinnacle of life. It is to that end that "How to Live Long and Like It", "The Longevity Diet" is presented here.

"Be such a man, and live such a life, that if every man were such as you, and every life a life like yours, this world would be God's paradise."

Phillips Brooks

"He who has wisdom possesses a blessing to bestow in his longevity."

Jim Heckathorn

"It is not the length of life but the depth of life."

Ralph Waldo Emerson

PART 1
Basis for Longevity

Chapter One
The History of Longevity

Biblical Times

The earliest references to longevity are found in the Holy Bible. In Genesis Chapter 5, a genealogy is given of ten men who lived an average of nine hundred years, the longest being Methuselah, who lived 969 years. After Noah, the life expectancy of man (often meaning men and women) descended rapidly to a maximum of about 120 years. This is consistent with Genesis 6:3, where God proclaims that the days of mortal man would be 120 years.

We may question why these early men lived so long. There are two factors that we may determine for this. The first is that when God created the earth, He made a perfect environment in which humans could live. Here He provided "every herb that yields seed which is on the face of the earth, and every tree whose fruit yields seed; to you it shall be for food – I have given every green herb for food" *(Gen.1:29-30)*. So there was an abundance of nourishing food growing naturally for the taking. (Note that meat was not originally included as a dietary item.) This food was undoubtedly eaten raw as they did not have the means to cook their food. It is quite possible that after the flood in the time of Noah these nourishing food supplies were not so available due to environmental changes. One can also speculate that there may have been a super food (perhaps an actual Tree of Life; a sign of continued life conditioned upon continual obedience) that disappeared from the earth at the time of the flood (Gen.2:9; 3:22). The longevity of these early people may also be attributed to God's Spirit dwelling with them to provide their longevity in

1

ways beyond their own "flesh". Examples of this are Enoch, who walked with God in such a pleasing manner that God took him, and Noah, who was obedient to build the ark although subjected to ridicule. These were not the only living men at the time, and nothing is said to indicate how long others lived.

The wide variety of healthful foods available to the people in Biblical times is confirmed by the many scripture references found in the Bible, a few of which are indicated here.

> "A land of wheat and barley, and vines and fig trees, and pomegranates, a land of olive oil and honey" (Deuteronomy 8:8).

In biblical times bread was considered to be so important that it was spoken of as "the staff of life". This was appropriate due to the great nutritional value to be found in these grains. Barley, along with potatoes and rice, is a balanced starch, rich in complex carbohydrates. Bread made from barley and wheat was the staple item in the diet. The bread was unleavened. In addition to being used for flour, the grain was frequently eaten raw or boiled and parched, or sometimes the ears were soaked and roasted. These grains were also used in many other ways such as soups and porridges.

The vines were grape vines. Grapes were eaten fresh, but more importantly they were used to make wine, which was a staple drink as water was often not available or not safe for drinking. Grapes were also dried for raisins. Fresh wine was simply grape juice, but it could not be kept long without fermenting. The fermentation process releases polyphenols which gives the wine an antibiotic activity that effectively kills germs. If drinking water made one sick, drinking wine was the cure. Of course, the wine was also intoxicating if not consumed in moderation; therefore, the scriptures contain warnings about drinking wine in excess (Ephesians 5:18). The many uses and benefits of grapes made them essential to the diet of the time.

There are so many passages in the Bible referring to olives that one cannot miss the importance of olive trees. The people found ways to incorporate olives or olive oil in nearly every meal. Olive oil was used not only nutritionally but also medicinally due to its healing properties. It was also used for cosmetics, rituals, and lamp fuel.

In Old Testament times honey was first available as wild honey which was collected from the bee's nests in holes in the ground, but later bee farming occurred. Honey was considered as a luxury as it was not so commonly available, but it was desired as a sweetener. The phrase "land of olive oil and honey" meant not only these but "all good things".

There were many kinds of fruits available to the people in biblical times. Most notably, in addition to grapes there were apples, pomegranates, and figs. The figs were eaten raw or were dried and pressed into cakes. It is also notable that there is no specific reference to apricots, except that in Proverbs 25:11 it says, "a word fitly spoken is like apples of gold" which likely refers to apricots. Apricots are one of the most common fruits in the Mediterranean world, which includes the Holy Land, so they certainly would have been an important item in the diet. The scarcity of references to vegetables indicates that they were not favored as food. This may have been because they had to be used fresh. Therefore, this vital source of vitamins and other nourishment was not fully utilized.

Another important reference elaborates further on the biblical foods;

> "...wheat and barley and flour and roasted grain and broad beans and lentils and parched grain; and honey and butter and sheep and curds of cattle they brought forward for David and the people that were with him to eat" (2 Samuel 17:28-29)

Broad beans and other legumes were easily cultivated by the crude methods available to early farmers, and they could be dried and stored for later use.

Meat was not a regular item in the biblical diet, especially in the earlier times; however, they may have hunted wild game when it was available. As humans became herdsmen, the most common meat was that of sheep and goats and sometimes, on very special occasions, a calf. A fatted calf was a calf that had been raised in a stall for such an occasion. The meat of the sheep was preferred over goat meat, but young goats were acceptable. Those living near the Sea of Galilee and the Jordan River were able to obtain fish, which became a frequent part of their diet. By New Testament times, fishing had become an important industry on the Sea of Galilee. There are also references to quail and fowl, most likely geese and wild ducks. The reference to the cock crowing indicates the presence of chickens. The eggs of these birds were also eaten.

The meaning of curds is somewhat indefinite, but it seems to refer to yogurt or cheeses which were known to be a part of their diet. These were made from goat milk, perhaps also sheep's or cow's milk, and were a good source of calcium and protein. Modern yogurt, due to its nutritional value and probiotics, is believed to contribute to longevity.

Other foods that contributed, more or less, depending upon location, to the diet in biblical times included almonds, pistachio nuts, onions, garlic, cucumbers, and melons (muskmelon). However, these foods were only available in some parts of the region

> "For the earth which drinks in the rain that often comes
> upon it, and bears herbs useful for those by whom it is
> cultivated, receives blessings from God" (Hebrews 6:7).

Herbs were cultivated for use as flavorings for food, and some herbs were also known to have medicinal value. These herbs included parsley, mint, coriander (today called cilantro), and hyssop, which was used for flavoring food and as a medicinal tea known to have cleansing properties.

We know that a wide variety of healthful foods existed for the people of biblical times, but not all foods were always available and affordable. It is notable that they apparently made little use of green vegetables, preferring grains (especially for bread), fruits including grapes (and its products), olive oil, nuts, meat, curds, and the other foods as available. Their diet was very healthful when a balanced diet was possible. We must be mindful that these people got a lot of exercise as the main means of getting around was by foot travel and most of their work was done by hand. Little is known about the longevity of the people in these later biblical times. Tradition has it that the apostle John lived to a very old age in Ephesus so a degree of longevity was possible. The bottom line here is that God provided everything we need for health and longevity. Dr. Lorraine Day, M.D. says, "You can't improve on God".

Hunza Valley, Pakistan

Over the years of recorded history it has been noted that there are an outstanding number of centenarians especially in some localized areas of the world. Outstanding among these are people of the Hunza Valley in the northern part of Pakistan near the China border. This valley, with an elevation of eight thousand feet, is surrounded by the Himalayan Mountains. The people who live in this valley are known for their friendliness and hospitality. Their literacy rate is about 90%.

The Hunza people are outstandingly free of disease, and this is believed to be due to their simple, healthy diet consisting of organically grown food including vegetables and fruits of apricots, apples, peaches, pears, cherries, mulberries, and grapes. Apricots particularly are a mainstay. The Hunza people eat them fresh and dry them in the sun for eating during the winter. They make apricot jam without sugar because of the natural sweetness of the fruit. The women hand grind the apricot pits with stone mortars to extract the oil, the uses of which include cooking, fuel, salad dressing and as a facial lotion. Their diet of organic vegetables and fruits provides an abundant amount of vitamins and other nutritional goodness.

Their liquid intake is from a wine that they make from red grapes, but of particular note is that they drink large amounts of a very special supply of pure water flowing from the glaciers in the mountains. This mineral rich milky colored water is called "Glacial Milk". This living water has been found to have a higher alkaline pH and an outstanding amount of active hydrogen, which creates very high antioxidant activity in the body. Some manufacturers have created machines that somewhat duplicate this water.

The Hunzas eat a bread called Chapatti Bread that is made fresh daily from stone-ground grains including wheat, barley, buckwheat, and millet. This delicious flat bread is unleavened and constitutes an important part of their diet.

The health and longevity of the Hunzas can be attributed in part to this diet and also to the healthy exercise they get every day which produces very strong bodies. Their normal daily activities include working outdoors in the fields and hiking 15 kilometers or more on mountain trails which are decidedly more rigorous than sidewalks. They also actively participate in volleyball played in the hot sun and an aggressively violent form of polo. Even the older men participate in these games. In winter, they sometimes break the ice to swim in the icy water of streams.

The result of the Hunza lifestyle is that they have strong bodies and experience almost no heart disease, cancer, bone, dental, or vision problems. They typically live to be 120-140 years of age. Men who are 110 can father children, and women who are 80 can conceive and bear children. A woman who is 80 years old may have the complexion, agility, and appearance of a 40 year old. While the Hunza lifestyle is in some respects more primitive than most would desire, it provides a very good example of the effects of lifestyle on longevity.

Okinawa, Japan

Another cultural group known to have perhaps the highest percentage of centenarians is the Japanese people on the island of Okinawa. On a percentage basis these people are noted for having perhaps the longest disability free life expectancy in the world. The average life expectancy is eighty-six for women and seventy-eight for men, but there are many exceptions. The prevalence of centenarians is approximately thirty-five for each 100,000 population. The Okinawans have kept strict census records since 1870 which verify their claims to longevity.

As these people get older, they remain in a very good state of mind and body. Centenarians are lean and energetic and, compared to Americans, they have a much lower risk of heart attack, stroke, cancer, osteoporosis, and dementia. Some who are in their nineties claim to maintain a healthy sex life.

They stay very active even in their senior years. Those 80-90 years old live like persons thirty years younger. Some who are one hundred years old are not yet thinking of retirement, but those who do, find ways to stay active. These activities frequently include gardening and selling some of their produce. They have hobbies, ride bicycles and motorcycles, practice karate, dance, and walk several kilometers on a daily basis. They also remain involved in social activities whereby they maintain a sense of community, and they sincerely maintain their spiritual side.

Scientific studies have revealed healthy hormone levels in these people. Their DHEA hormone levels decrease more slowly, so they age more slowly. Compared to Americans, they also have higher levels of hormones (testosterone in men and estrogen in women) which help to maintain their vitality. They also have fewer free radicals in their bodies.

This long, healthy life expectation is attributed to their diet and exercise. They eat more tofu and soy than is consumed in any other part of the world. A typical meal consists of a bowl of cooked food and a fruit. They consume a lot of vegetables, including sweet potatoes, which are a staple, and seaweed. The seaweed consumed is a very nutritious super food containing all of the amino acids along with many vitamins, minerals, proteins, and other essential nutrients. Seaweed is harvested in many parts of the world, but Okinawans consume the most. Where it is not available they can obtain it as a food supplement. Portions of fish and pork are eaten weekly. Irregularly they eat dairy products. Their average daily intake may consist of seven portions of vegetables and fruit, seven of whole grains, and two of soy products. Although this may seem like a lot, the portions are small as they try to keep their total intake to about 1,200 calories per day. They control their intake by eating from a small bowl or plate, and they practice eating only until they are about eighty percent full. Their diet is low in fat, salt, and sugar. When they cook pork, they boil it to remove the fat. Their principle beverage is tea. They drink copious amounts of turmeric tea daily. They also favor sanpin tea, which is an antioxidant rich form of green tea.

About thirty percent of their longevity may be attributed to the genes they inherit, but this is not the most important factor. When about 100,000 Okinawans moved to Brazil and their young people adopted the local diet around military bases that consisted largely of pizza and fast foods, it was found that their health and life expectancy decreased. Other studies have revealed that when Okinawans consume American-style fast foods, their health and longevity suffers.

Okinawans are a positive people who live lives that are relatively stress free. They have skills to cope well with their life situations. They maintain a good sense of meaning and purpose. When they are aged, eighty percent continue to live independently in their own homes. They have close bonds with family, so that the younger generations are very respectful and supportive of their parents and grandparents. Although the children may move away from their parents, they take responsibility to maintain close contacts. Especially on festive occasions, they gather in family groups for the celebration. There is also a great sense of community among neighbors and friends whereby they demonstrate mutual care and assistance to attend to the needs of their fellowman.

The Okinawans demonstrate that living a healthy lifestyle is the key to living a longer, happier and disease free life, or as we say, they live long and live well.

Ikaria, Italy

We now turn our focus on two locations in the Mediterranean area. The first of these is Ikaria (sometimes Icaria), which is a Greek island in the Aegean Sea having an area of one hundred square miles. The island is very mountainous and features luxurious oak and pine forests and many streams and ponds, some of which are radon active and are claimed to be healthful to bathers.

There are approximately 8300 residents on the island. It is outstanding that one out of three of these people is ninety years of age or older. They are very healthy, having twenty percent less cancer than Americans and about half as much heart disease and very little diabetes. Alzheimer's disease (dementia) is practically unknown there. The residents are known for their unhurried, low-stress lifestyle; in which they live like there is always tomorrow. They take their time in all that they do and most days take time for a thirty to forty-five minute nap. Two of the secrets of their longevity must be avoiding stress and getting plenty of rest.

The diet of these people is a modified Mediterranean diet consisting of vegetables, fruit, beans, legumes, potatoes, whole grains, meat (mostly fish), and olive oil. The principle part of their daily meal is vegetables. They raise gardens without using chemicals, so their produce is organic. At least 70 varieties of wild greens grow in the fields and along the roadsides and are gathered for eating. Some of these have ten times more anti-oxidants than wine. Their honey is known to have anticancer, antibacterial, and anti-inflammatory properties. Although they use olive oil in cooking, they will sprinkle a little more on their food before they eat.

There are an estimated 35,000 goats on the island, so it is no surprise that they drink much goat milk. This milk is known to be rich in L-tryptophan which is heart-healthy. They also consume much herbal tea, mainly a local mint tea and chamomile. They also drink a rich wine that is locally made.

These people get a lot of exercise from their daily activities since they walk rather than depending upon other transportation. There is a bus line that operates on the island that can be used when traveling the longer distances between cities.

The Icarians are very religious and faithfully attend church services and religious festivals and observances. They are very social, always having time to visit with friends. They also have very strong family ties.

Assessing the reasons for the longevity of the Ikarians, it seems apparent that it is not only attributed to diet but also to their lifestyle.

Ovodda, Sardinia

The second Mediterranean area that we are focusing on is the community of Ovodda on the island of Sardinia. This island, 150 miles west of mainland Italy, has an area of 9,301 square miles, making it the second largest of the Italian islands. Ovodda is located in a mountainous area in the central part of Sardinia. It is an agricultural area primarily producing sheep, goats, wheat, grapes, and olives.

The population of Ovodda is approximately 1,665, and there are at any time five to seven centenarians. An unusual feature of their longevity is that, whereas women are usually more long-lived, here the men live as long as the women.

The residents of this community eat a somewhat typical Mediterranean diet except that they eat more meat than is usual in other places on the island. The meat is usually that of the goats and sheep that they raise. A staple is bread, homemade with barley or bran flour and potatoes. Other foods are fava beans, zucchini, tomatoes, potatoes, onions, eggplant, and pecorino cheese which is made from sheep milk. They drink goat and sheep milk and a lot of red wine. Sardinians are known to eat only two meals each day. Breakfast may be only goat's milk. Dinner in Ovodda is a larger meal consisting of meat and vegetables.

Ovodda differs from the other areas we have considered in that genetics seem to play a larger role in their longevity. Most of the residents are descended from a few early families that settled there. As they are somewhat isolated in the mountains, the families have intermarried. The result of this inbreeding is that it seems to have caused a gene expression that has contributed in great measure to their longevity.

These people get plenty of exercise from their daily activities. They work hard all of their lives and walk about five miles each day. This helps them to stay lean and healthy.

The residents of this community are of the Roman Catholic faith. They enjoy their festivals, times of fellowship, and getting together for parties. It seems that their lives are lived with little stress. While genetics are an important factor in the longevity of the Ovoddans, their variety of the Mediterranean diet and their lifestyle are also important features contributing to their longevity.

The United States

Over the last one hundred years, we have come a long way toward increasing the longevity of our people. In the year 1900, the incidence of centenarians in the United States was one for every 10,000 population. Current statistics indicate one per 4,400 of population. On September 1, 2010, the number of centenarians in the U.S. was calculated to be 70,490, which is the greatest of any nation in the world. This great number may be credited partly to our large population and to improvements in health care. The current life expectancy in the U.S. is seventy-six years for men and eighty-one years for women. The great number of centenarians is proof that it is very possible to exceed the average.

In their book "121 Ways to Live 121 Years"[1] (p.129) Dr. Ronald Klatz and Dr. Robert Goldman say, "We may consider the years 2006 through 2029 collectively as a Bridge to Practical Immortality, during which science will amass key knowledge in biomedical technologies that will enable us 150+ year-long lifespans;" however, in the absence of these biomedical technologies people have been finding ways to extend their lifespans past the age of one hundred years. This is largely due to our own awareness and efforts to take better care of ourselves with our way of life along with the assistance of improved health care.

While some Americans are living longer than ever, the statistics indicate that, on a worldwide basis, we have been surpassed by thirty-six other nations that have made gains in their life expectancy. One of the reasons for this is that we have a weight problem. Just look around and notice the people you see wherever you go. Over sixty-seven percent of Americans are overweight, and over thirty percent of these are actually obese. Up to a third, or more, of the decrease in overall longevity may be attributed to obesity. The risks of obesity are revealed in diabetes, stroke, and heart disease. The problem is due to lifestyle choices. Paul Terry, an assistant professor of epidemiology at Emory University in Atlanta, Georgia, has said, "We have the luxury of choosing a bad lifestyle as opposed to having one imposed on us by hard times."

A new report released by the National Research Council indicates that smoking tobacco products is another serious problem that negatively affects our national life expectancy. Currently twenty percent of Americans are smokers, whereas a few decades ago in 1960 more than forty percent of adults were smokers. The effects are becoming evident as these smokers grow older. Studies made in the past have predicted that smoking would shorten a person's lifespan. The longer a person smokes and the greater the indulgence, the more serious the negative effect will be on her or his lifespan. The bright spots here are that the incidence of smoking has decreased and that medical science has improved the treatment of cancers, heart problems, and other ailments caused by this habit. It is to be noted that the effects of inhaling secondhand smoke are also a part of the smoking problem.

A third aspect of our lifestyle problem is that we have adopted a sedentary lifestyle. Our children are spending more time in front of the television and playing computer games instead of being outdoors, running, or playing sports to burn calories. Even adults have chosen activities that are more sedentary. Many eat their meals in front of the television and often spend their evenings watching television, using a computer or perhaps reading. We sit to busy ourselves with various hobbies. There is a need to balance our lifestyle to provide more activity to stimulate healthy blood circulation throughout the body. One of the authors of the National Research Council study on longevity, Samuel Preston, a demographer at the University of Pennsylvania, has stated that the overall physical and mental wellness of Americans "is relatively poor".

In the United States, our ethnic backgrounds, environments, education, and ways of life are very diverse; however, some interesting features have been noticed. Many centenarians are healthy, alert, and agile, enabling them to continue to live in their own homes. They are people who have done something right to enable them to overcome the maladies, diseases, and mental decline that befall so many.

It has been noted that the people in Minnesota and the upper Great Plains states are setting records for living a few years longer than people in other parts of the United States, but there is no criterion to explain this. On the other hand, there is a group of people at Loma Linda in Southern California that from the onset of their organization has purposefully designed a lifestyle that is enabling them to live long and live well. These people are of the Seventh-Day Adventists (SDA) faith, and, although we are looking at them in Loma Linda, they exist all over the United States and in many other world areas. Wherever you find them, they teach their people to practice the same lifestyle.

For the SDA longevity is a matter of the way they interpret the teachings of the Bible and apply them to their lives in these modern times. Their vegetarian dietary lifestyle is because of their belief in the holistic nature of humankind. They follow the scriptural admonition, "Therefore whether you eat or drink, or whatever you do, do all to the glory of God" (1 Cor. 10:31 NKJV). They believe that it is dishonoring to God to put anything into their bodies that does not have a sound nutritional benefit to preserve the health of the body, mind and spirit.

Their position statement on vegetarian diets states, "The vegetarian diet recommended by the SDA includes the generous use of whole grain breads, cereals and pastas, a liberal use of fresh vegetables and fruits, a moderate use of legumes, nuts, seeds. It can also include low fat dairy products such as milk, yogurt, cheeses and eggs. It is best to avoid high saturated fat and cholesterol foods such as beef, pork, chicken, fish and seafood. Coffee, tea, and alcoholic beverages provide few nutrients and may interfere with the absorption of essential nutrients."

This is what they state and is not necessarily factual. Actually there appear to be some inconsistencies in it. Their dietary recommendations have varied over the more than 130 years since their beginning, and not all SDA members follow the guideline to the same degree or even perhaps at all. Some are more strictly vegan, and some eat more meat. The temptations of processed and fast foods are always before them and are especially tempting to the younger generation. Nevertheless, they have an outstanding number of seniors that are living longer than the common lifespan of Americans and are not only living longer but living well. According to studies from the 1970's and 1980's, they have fifty percent less risk of heart disease, certain types of cancers, strokes, and diabetes. Recent SDA data suggests that vegetarian men under forty can expect to live more than eight years longer and women more than seven years longer than the general population.

In addition to their suggested diet, the SDA recommend that their people maintain a healthy exercise program and abstain from using tobacco products, alcoholic beverages, and drugs.

Loma Linda is located in a large valley and is surrounded by many other cities within fifty miles that together form a very large metropolis. It has been noted that although the air quality in the Loma Linda area is very poor, due to smog and inversions that hold the bad air down in their valley, the negative effect on health is uncertain, This may be because they live and work indoors and many of their exercise and recreational facilities are also indoors at the times when the air quality is worst. Another environmental problem is that their water supply, which comes from underground wells, is contaminated with industrial pollutants that get into the aquifer. Although it is approved for consumption, it leaves much to be desired.

"Only I can change my life. No one can do it for me."
Carol Burnett

"Happiness is not a destination. It is a method of life."
Burton Hills

"May you live all the days of your life."
Jonathan Swift

Chapter Two
Centenarian and Nearly Centenarian Stories

The information for the following biographies was obtained by this author, and/or, by another interviewer, as indicated, who kindly shared the information. The interviews were conducted either face-to-face, by phone, or in writing with the individual, or a next of kin.

Gladys Burril:

Ansel Oliver, a Seventh-Day Adventist assistant director for news, reported an outstanding feat of a ninety-two year old SDA lady. Gladys Burrill has a home in Prospect, Oregon and also one in Honolulu, Hawaii. Burrill, who is a widow, is the mother of five, and has outlived a son who died in 1985.

Over the past years she has power walked in marathons several times. On December 12, 2010, she power walked the Honolulu Marathon, an official twenty-six mile race, finishing in nine hours and fifty-three minutes. If her time is approved by the Guinness Book of world records it will be a new world record.

Her time might have been better had she not stopped to pray a few hundred yards from the finish. "I thought my life would change once I crossed that line. I knew some people needed encouragement, so I thought that was very important," Burrill said.

Burrill has had to overcome several difficulties in her life. Her father died on her second birthday, so she was raised on their farm by her mother.

When she was eleven years old, she contracted polio but recovered from that. Then there have been the deaths of her family members. Life, like a marathon, requires "perseverance, strength, courage . . . You just have to keep going," Burrill said.

Adventure and exercise have helped her deal with stress and grief throughout her life. "Sometimes I go out (walking) with the weight of the world on my shoulders and come back feeling so strong and renewed," she says.

Burrill walks thirty to fifty miles every week, usually with a training partner. She has always been athletic. She has also been an airplane pilot and a mountain climber.

When asked for advice on fitness, she keeps it simple, "Eat healthy and exercise. So many young people don't realize the importance of exercise. Just put one foot in front of the other", she said. She has never used alcohol or tobacco and eats a healthy diet that is mostly vegetarian.

Used by permission of Ansel Oliver and Adventists News Network, Silver Spring, MD 20904

* * * * *

Agnes Loreen Dinwiddie:

At 109 years of age, Loreen Dinwiddie was just one year shy of being a super-centenarian (110 years or older) when she died on August 25, 2012. Loreen was born February 03, 1903. She received some notoriety when she was interviewed by a Portland, Oregon KGW–TV news anchor on her 108th birthday. Loreen, formerly of Gresham, resided at Cherry Blossom Cottage in southeast Portland for several years just prior to her death. When she was interviewed the TV reporter commented that her appearance was amazing for her age. Her skin was clear and radiant with hardly any wrinkles that a lady of her age might be expected to have. Her mind was sharp, and she spoke eloquently.

Loreen, whose maiden name was Johnson, grew up as one of a large family, living on a farm near Sequim, WA. Life on the farm necessitated a lot of hard work for her. After graduation from high school, she attended

Walla Walla College, working for ten cents per hour to get by. During her lifetime, she has lived in Washington, California, Oregon, and Montana. She was married two times. Her first husband, whom she met at Walla Walla College, was Frank W. Stunenberg, the youngest son of former Idaho Governor Frank Steunenberg who was murdered in 1905 by Harry Orchard. This marriage was not successful and he divorced her. She later married a Seventh-Day Adventist pastor, Howard Dinwiddie, who preceded her in death. During her working years, she was employed as an office worker. Her life always involved a lot of hard work, but her disposition was such that she was always able to persevere through the difficulties of her life.

Loreen had macular degeneration and had not been able to read for over two years. She lived by herself until June 1, 2006. The evening just prior to that, she fell off of her couch and laid on the floor, unable to reach her phone some six feet away. She endured until a nurse found her the following morning. She had dislocated her left shoulder and broken her upper arm. She had suffered a heart attack either before or after the fall.

Until this time she was self-sufficient, cooking three meals each day and taking the weekly shopping bus for groceries. She lived in the Village Retirement Center (Gresham) for over thirty years, where she had a garden plot in which she raised vegetables for over twenty years. After that she had a raised bed behind her apartment for a few vegetables and raspberry plants. She had pneumonia but recovered well and since then was able to go to the dining room for her meals.

Loreen obviously inherited some longevity genes that aided her in overcoming the hardships of her life. Her mother and father, two sisters, and a brother all lived to be ninety to one hundred years of age. Her mother lived to be nearly one hundred years old. Loreen's long life ended as the result of dementia due to cerebrovascular disease.

She was a faithful life-long member of the Seventh-Day Adventists Church (SDA). She attributed her longevity to adhering to the church's dietary instruction. She was a strict vegan, who ate no meat whatsoever, for approximately thirty-five years. In an interview she said that her diet had kept her feeling wonderful all the years of her life. She daily took some vitamins, especially a multiple vitamin, along with vitamins C and E. When she felt that she may get a cold, she took goldenseal and echinacea. During her latter years she spent a lot of time resting since she was experiencing some difficulty with her eyes. She had two daughters and one step-daughter. As only one of these lived very near, her fellowship was mostly with others who lived in the retirement center.

Appreciation is extended to Alice Willoughby, daughter of Loreen, for providing information and for permission to use it in this biography.

* * * * *

Iola Hankins:

Iola Hankins is a centenarian lady living in Bonanza, Oregon. She devoted most of her life to being a farmer's wife on a farm about three miles out of town. Now a widow, she moved into town in 2009 where she has lived with her son and his wife. She has persevered to live a long life in spite of hardships, some illness and much hard work.

Iola Hankins was born on November 08,1910. Her maiden name was Davison. Although she is now a centenarian approaching 104 years of age, she is pretty spry for her age. Rather than needing a caregiver, she has helped to care for her diabetic son who died in 2013. She has continued to live with her daughter-in-law.

Iola was born at Dickey, North Dakota. After her parents divorced she lived with her mother at Carson, North Dakota where her mother had a café for awhile. They later moved to Thunder Hawk, South Dakota. She only got an eighth grade education as her dad moved so often. When she was thirteen years old she was very ill with a ruptured appendix which put her in the hospital for fifty-eight days. She said. "If it weren't for praying people she would not be here." When she was nineteen years old she moved to Oregon with her mother. There she worked as a milk maid which she found to be hard work.

In 1931 she married Lloyd Hankins and they moved to a run-down farm near Bonanza, Oregon. Iola commented that at that time there were few roads and no telephones there. She found that nothing came easy as life on the farm was also hard work.

One thing readily noticeable about Iola is that she is a staunch

Christian. She attends church services regularly, reads her Bible, and attends two Bible studies every week. She still drives her car locally to get to these activities which also provide her with fellowship opportunities outside of the home.

That she is highly regarded in the community is attested to by the fact that she has twice been chosen to be the Grand Marshall in a local celebration which gave her prominence in the community's parade.

Hankins is a typical old-fashioned lady who engages in common home skills including sewing and quilting. Although she enjoys cooking, over the past fifteen years she has become more health conscious and eats a healthy diet consisting of vegetables, whole grains, some fruit, and chicken. Although she likes to eat raw foods, her dentures make chewing a bit difficult. She is allergic to milk, so she avoids dairy products and eats only a few sweets. She said that she takes vitamins daily and "a good dose of God" to keep her going.

Stresses in her life, in addition to her childhood illness were, the loss of her husband, her son, and she had to face the dread of cancer in 1984. She went through surgery courageously and has been free of the disease since then. Her only health problem now is that she has to watch her blood pressure. If you were to meet Iola face-to-face you would imagine her to be much younger than her actual age. Although she has white hair, she has a very nice complexion with only a few light wrinkles and a very pleasant smile.

When asked what advice she would give to others who desire to live a good long life, Iola readily replied, "Live right, eat right, and love the Lord."

* * * * *

Fulsom "Charles" Scrivner:

This outstanding centenarian man was a personal friend of this author. Mr. Scrivner was called "Chief" by many friends because of his Chickasaw heritage derived from his mother, who was half Chickasaw. His father was German. His wife, Fern, and others referred to him as Charles. While in college he gave himself the name "Charles" preferring that to Fulsom.

"Chief" lived to be 102 years old. He was born in Sulphur, Oklahoma on July 18, 1910. He had a twin brother that died when seventy-five years of age. He was married seventy-three years to Fern, a retired teacher, who was in her mid-nineties when he went to be with the Lord. Their home for their retirement years was in in Nampa, Idaho.

Charles studied at Oklahoma University, The University of New Mexico, and Pasadena College. He earned a Master's Degree in School Administration and was an ordained minister who did missionary work among the American Indians. He was also occupied as an educator in public and private secondary schools and at an Indian Bible college. For a time, he found employment in law enforcement, but ministry was his special calling. Charles was very active all of his life, and, as a missionary working with Indian people, he planted and built several churches. While working on one of these projects when he was sixty-five, he got tuberculosis. Some others who also contracted it were sent home to die. With rest, some care, and the support of his strong immune system, Charles was able to overcome the TB, and, to the amazement of his doctor, his lung completely healed itself.

His daughter, Janice Miller, commented that "Dad's hard work in ministry was a blessing and joy to him. I never once heard him complain of it or the people of whom he loved so deeply, the American Indians. Dad was part Chickasaw from Oklahoma; to see him talk and move his hands in such a way you'd think he was full blood and raised on the reservation. He was God's man "for such a time as this" to the people he served. In his early years of ministry, family and marriage they worked and lived in California, Arizona and New Mexico. He worked very hard teaching, building and preaching. Later on, he enjoyed studying and authoring books about different tribes."

He has written several books about American Indians including *The Mohave People (1970), The Beautiful Paiute Girl (1996),* and *The Golden Cities of Cibola (a children's story).* His last book, *Early Chickasaws: Profile of Courage,* was published in 2005 when he was 95 years old. These can be found on the internet.

Until just two years prior to his death Charles and Fern lived in their own home with the help of caregivers that came in for a few hours each day. While in their home Fern had suffered a mild stroke but recovered nicely. She has had two hip replacements but manages to keep going. For many years, Charles would go for long walks carrying a cane, only to fend-off any troublesome dogs. He exercised daily for thirty minutes, using his treadmill, riding his stationary bike, and doing other arm and body exercises. Until he was 101 years old he continued to drive his automobile for distances not exceeding five miles due to a medication he was taking that could cause dizziness. However, when he was ninety-two years old he drove 270 miles, on two occasions, to my home to help me pour concrete. In all of his years of driving he never had an accident. He had a mild stroke a couple years prior to his death.

One reason he gave for his longevity is that, throughout his lifetime, he practiced clean habits. He never used tobacco, didn't consumed any alcoholic beverages, or use any drugs.

The Scrivners, who were Nazarenes, enjoyed their togetherness. They began their day with a devotional time at their kitchen table. They considered this to be a very special time for them. Until shortly before his illness leading to death, they attended church very regularly. For several years, he attended a Men's Bible Study until the leader was unable to continue. In 2011 he said that he had lost ten pounds in twenty years, never gaining it back. This is attributed to eating a balanced diet consisting of a special white bread, potatoes, beans, whole grains, and vegetables. Sometimes they included chicken. They didn't use salt but did like to put sugar on their cereal. They didn't eat very many sweets but did treat themselves at times to a piece of pie. At mealtimes, they became accustomed to eating small portions. In addition to water, they drank coffee, orange juice, and some milk. Charles did, however, confess that he liked to go to McDonald's to have a double hamburger and a soda for lunch while enjoying some fellowship. His disposition was to always be cheerful.

Of their family life, Janice, commented, "Some of my fondest memories of Dad are our long drives thru the countryside when he would talk about all kinds of topics. When going thru the desert he would speak of the different rock formations. I loved that! You could ask him anything and if he didn't know the answer, he would go find it and get back to you on it. In the latter years, not so long ago, after dinner we'd all linger and talk about matters of the heart. His respect and love for the Lord reflected in his prayers, when he spoke with such honor to Him."

The Scrivners took great interest in their family consisting of two daughters and a son, their grandchildren and also to their many friends. The purpose of his life was to love and serve God and to share that love among his family and friends. At 101 years of age he said that he wanted to live longer to share love and togetherness with Fern. Love is what has motivated and kept him going. The Bible says, "It is not good that man should be alone" (Gen.2:18). Charles and Fern Scrivner have given evidence of the benefits of togetherness. They gave us something to aspire to. Charles went to his eternal reward on October 21, 2012 at the age of 102.

* * * * *

George Beverly Shea:

Here is a man who truly enjoyed living. Bev Shea was born on February 1, 1909 in Winchester, Ontario, Canada. His father, Rev. Adam J. Shea, who was a Wesleyan Methodist pastor, taught him to play the violin, and his mother, Erma, taught him to play the piano and organ. He got his start as a baritone singer by singing in his father's church and at religious meetings in the Ottawa Valley. Music uplifted his heart and soul throughout his lifetime.

While he grew up with Christian influence and became a Christian believer at the early age of five or six years, he later really made a full commitment at the age of eighteen, when he was not feeling too spiritual. His dad was pastor of a church in Ottawa, and the church was having a week-long "special effort" to win souls. On Friday evening, his father came down from the pulpit, tenderly laid his hand on Bev's shoulder and whispered, "I think tonight might be the night, son, when you come back to the Lord." That night Bev Shea made a final commitment to the Lord, from which he never deviated or doubted God's grace.

Bev is known for writing the music and for singing "I'd Rather Have Jesus". In the February 2009 issue of the Decision magazine, he tells how he happened to do this. "At the age of twenty-three, I was living at home with my parents, continuing to work at Mutual Life Insurance and studying voice with Manley Price Boone, traveling by subway and the Hudson River ferry every day. Going to the piano one Sunday morning, I found a poem waiting for me there. I recognized my mother's handwriting. She had copied the words of a poem by Rhea F. Miller, knowing her son would read the beautiful message, which speaks of choice. As I read these precious words: "I'd rather have Jesus than men's applause; I'd rather be faithful to His dear cause," I found myself singing the words in a melody that expressed the feeling of my heart. What a joy it was to sing with fervent voice in the key of b-flat:

"Than to be the king of a vast domain
Or be held in sin's dread sway,
I'd rather have Jesus than anything
This world affords today."

Soon my mother's arms were around my shoulders. She had been in the next room having her devotions and now, joining me at the piano, there were tears in her eyes. She knew the words were having the desired effect – they were speaking to me about life's choices."[2]

Bev Shea embarked upon his lifetime calling when a young evangelist, Billy Graham, invited him to join with him in his ministry, the Billy Graham Crusade. Joining in this ministry, he sang his first song at a crusade in Charlotte, NC on a November night, and continued in this role for decades.

In his autobiography, *Just As I Am*, Billy Graham wrote, "Bev Shea was the very first person I asked to join me in evangelism. He was well known in the Midwest, but at the same time he was humble; he couldn't say no, even to a Fuller Brush salesman! It was God who brought us together. Bev will always be remembered as 'America's beloved Gospel singer,' whose rich bass baritone voice has touched the hearts of millions in our Crusades and through his sixty-five recordings; one of them, 'Song's of the Southlands,' was awarded a Grammy."

On the occasion of Bev's one-hundreth birthday in February 2009, Decision magazine quoted long-time Billy Graham associate, Cliff Barrows, as saying, "We always knew that when Bev sang before Mr. Graham preached, the Spirit of God would override anything that had been said, sung, or done, and would prepare the people for the preaching of the word."

Bev Shea married his childhood sweetheart, Erma Scharfe, and they had a son and a daughter, both of whom accepted Christ as their Savior at early ages in Billy Graham Crusades. The most grievous and stressful time of Bev's life was when Erma passed away in 1976 after an extended illness. For ten long years, Bev continued on alone. His loneliness touched the hearts of his friends Billy and Ruth Graham. In his autobiography Mr. Graham says, "After repeated nudging by team members [meaning Billy and Ruth], Bev began to date one of the receptionists in our Montreat office. Karlene and Bev were married in 1985 (December 19) in a candlelight ceremony in our home and now live only a mile from us."[3] Bev commented that it has been years of married bliss.

We wonder why some people live so long. Bev's mother lived to be ninety years old, having died in 1971, so it seems that perhaps she passed on to him some longevity genes. Bev has had one major health problem with his heart in 1996, but afterward regained and maintained good health.

He ate a healthy diet consisting of vegetables and fruit including raw fruit and salads, whole grains, some dairy products, meat (but no red meat), and some sweets. He got exercise by walking but in his later years no longer drove a vehicle. He got out and around a lot for a person of his age but was no longer was able to attend church regularly. He read his Bible and other literature daily and had prayer times with his wife. He had good times of fellowship with his family and friends. Throughout his lifetime he enjoyed playing his organ and piano and singing the old hymns and gospel songs that were so much a part of his life.

In 1996 he had the privilege of singing at a ceremony where Ruth and Billy Graham were honored with the Congressional Gold Medal. In his lifetime, he was inducted into the Gospel Music Association Gospel Music Hall of Fame and the National Religious Broadcasters Hall of Fame, and was awarded two honorary doctorates. In February 2011, he was honored by the awarding of the GRAMMY Lifetime Achievement Award.

When asked what advice he would give to others who aspire to live a good long life, he responded, "To know Jesus as Savior". George Beverly Shea was a good example of what God can do with a life that is given over to the Lord. "Singing (he went) along life's way, praising the Lord, praising the Lord". At the age of 104, Bev Shea went to be with his Lord on April 16, 2013.

* * * * *

George Vrieling:

Born at Manhattan, Montana, on September 30, 1905, George Vrieling was 103 years old when he died on December 14, 2008. George was the son of Dutch immigrant farmers. When George struck out on his own, he moved around a bit before deciding to settle in the Grangeville, Idaho area. On November 1, 1927, he married Tena Workman. When the Great Depression of the 1930's came upon the nation George was hard pressed to survive. He and Tena went to Everett, Washington, where he worked for a little less than a year before coming back to Idaho determined to tough it out. When he had a God-given opportunity to buy a 160 acre farm near Harpster, Idaho, he acted on his faith in God to buy it. There he and Tena worked hard, using all of their initiative, ingenuity and resourcefulness to achieve success and rear five children. They raised a good garden every year and always had a few cows, a large flock of chickens, a small flock of sheep, and a couple pigs which he butchered for meat. They always had plenty to eat and to preserve, and enough milk and eggs to sell the surplus, which steadily added to their income.

George was always a good neighbor. Over the years, he would trade labor with his neighboring farmers. If someone needed a fence or a barn built, they would all get together to get the job done. If a neighbor got burned out, George was one of the first there to offer assistance, giving whatever was necessary without any thought of getting any return. He was very honest in all of his dealings being conscientious to promptly pay everything he owed to anyone.

George always enjoyed the fellowship and support of his close-knit, loving family, and when Tena died on September 16, 1973, George sensed a great loss. With his dear helpmate, Tena, deceased and the children all out on their own, George, now 69 years old, decided, not to retire, but to scale down on his farming. He sold his 160 acre farm in 1974 and purchased a 40 acre farm at the edge of Grangeville, where he was closer to some of his family.

Still George sensed loneliness and the need for a helpmate. To resolve his problem, he placed an advertisement in the "Rural Light", a small publication of the local rural electric company. In the advertisement he expressed an interest in having a female pen pal. A widowed lady named Beulah, seeing the ad, thought it seemed o.k., but had no thought of being anything more than a pen pal. As they wrote to each other, they became deeply interested in their budding friendship and soon decided to get together. About four months from the start, they were married on March 2, 1976, and Beulah moved onto the farm, near Grangeville, with George. In 2006, with Beulah beginning to have serious problems with her mobility, they moved into the Meadowlark retirement home, in Grangeville, where they could have some assistance.

After George and Beulah were married, they modified their diet some by limiting meat except for chicken, but they always had vegetables, fruit, whole grains, milk, and eggs. They also took a multiple vitamin tablet and vitamin C. daily.

The hallmark of George's life was a love for God and for the Bible. This was instilled in him as a child, and he nurtured it throughout his lifetime by reading the Bible daily, praying to his Lord, and having family devotions. In our interview Beulah said, "George had a lot of faith and loved to read the Bible." It was a heritage that he passed along to his children. He was a faithful member of the Christian Reformed Church and attended regularly. Beulah liked the Church of the Nazarene, so sometimes they would attend both, but as they got older they mostly attended the Church of the Nazarene.

George was always quite healthy; never having any serious illness up to the day he died. The only physical problem that he had was some difficulty with hearing. When friends would ask George about the secret reason for his longevity he would always reply, "Just keep going."

Beulah, who was born on March 30, 1915 in Minnesota, at the time of this writing, was 96 and continued to live at the Meadowlark. She was very alert and enjoyed reading to help pass the time. Her longevity was possibly partly due to genes passed down from her mother, who lived to be 99 years old. Beulah had been widowed and had three adult children when she and George met. During their years together, she and George had a loving relationship in which they were very considerate of each other's needs. Beulah passed away in January 2012.

* * * * *

Nola Ochs:

Here is a lady that anyone must surely admire. In 2010, at the age of 98, Nola Ochs graduated from Fort Hays State University at Hays, Kansas, which earned her a place in the Guinness Book of Records as the oldest person in the world to ever graduate from a college. Education has always been a foremost interest in Nola's life. Her graduation was a climatic point in that interest. When Nola walked across the stage to receive her diploma, she was accompanied by her granddaughter, Alexandra Ochs, who was also graduating. As she received her diploma (and a kiss on the cheek) from Kansas Governor Kathleen Sebelius, the audience in, filled to capacity, Gross Memorial Coliseum, rose to their feet to cheer her for her outstanding accomplishment. Her family were all present sporting "Nola's #1 Fans" T-shirts. She was recognized by the Associated Press and numerous radio shows, and even received a telephone greeting from BBS Global News in London. She later appeared on the Jay Leno T.V. show. Previous to her graduation, she was accompanied by her university adviser, Joleen Briggs, to a day-long Women's Leadership Conference where she was honored as Kansas Woman of the Year for 2007.

Nola's love for learning began in 1927 when she taught in a one room Hodgeman County rural school where she taught all eight grades. Lola commented, "At that time we could take a teaching examination out of Topeka, and if we passed we could teach." While teaching, she took her first college classes at Fort Hays Teachers College in 1930 with the motivation to further her teaching certificate. Her teaching career, however, was cut short when she decided to get married. Nola continued to explain, "At that time they would not allow a married woman to teach, because they didn't want a pregnant teacher in the school room. It was understood when we started to teach that if we got married we could no longer teach." While Nola enjoyed teaching and would have liked to continue in the profession, Vernon Ochs, with his 1929 Model A Ford coupe, won her over, and they were married.

Although education has been a great interest in Nola's life, she says, "I thoroughly enjoyed being a wife and the mother to my four sons. My one claim to fame has been being the mother of Vernon Ochs four sons. Everything else has just been a pastime." One of the blessings of teaching is seeing the results as the former students grow older and take their places in life. Nola said she 'thoroughly enjoyed watching her former students grow up to become fine citizens, good parents and good neighbors." However, Nola's family interest has eclipsed her educational and professional satisfaction. Her family has grown to include 13 grandchildren and 15 great grandchildren, in all of whom she takes great pride. Nola says her purpose in life now is "to encourage her grandchildren to seek higher education." She is setting the example for them.

Nola was born in Illinois on November 22, 1911 and moved with her family in 1928 to a farm near Jetmore, Kansas. Vernon's mother and sister were organizing a Sunday School at the schoolhouse, and Vernon, with his Ford coupe, provided transportation for Nola and her sister. Thus a budding romance began. Nola and Vernon went together for over three years before they decided to get married.

Although Nola's educational interests were sidetracked for several years, she still yearned for learning situations. She commented, "I started taking college classes at Dodge City Community College in 1977, because I wanted to find a way to fill my time after my husband died." Although her family was great she wanted more activity to fill her days. "I saw a tennis class listed on a schedule from the college. It was in the summertime, and I liked playing tennis when I was younger, so I enrolled in the class."

At that time, Nola had no thought of getting a degree, but rather of filling her time by being in learning situations. She continued, "After that I enrolled in an Agri-business course, and then I just kept adding classes in general studies. I never worried about getting a degree, I only took classes that I was interested in, and I enjoyed them all." After she was told by a professor at Dodge City that she lacked only one class for an associate's degree she got the motivation to seriously pursue an educational degree. The next spring she decided to attend Fort Hays State University (FHSU) because it was the nearest four–year college to her home in Jetmore.

Nola admitted that being a student at her age had some drawbacks that she had to overcome. "Physically, I can't hear as well as other traditional students, so the university let me sit at the front of the class so I could hear my instructors. Since that is where I would rather sit anyway. I enjoyed that. I read slower than I used to and sometimes I have to read material twice to get its full meaning, but I keep on working until I got the full meaning. . . I've worked like a beaver; but that's what I came here for. It was a lot of reading and a lot of writing. I knew when I came here that it would be mostly study, but I study diligently so that wasn't a problem." At the graduation Kansas Board of Regents member Dan Lykins commented, "Follow (in) the footsteps of people like Nola ... never give up!"

Getting around the large campus was another problem as parking spaces convenient to her classes were sometimes difficult to find. So that she would not have to walk so far lugging her heavy books the university granted her a special parking permit which granted her special permission to park in any available space, even in spots designated "No Parking". She really appreciated the thoughtfulness of this assistance.

Nola explained her plan to get a parking pass when she moved from her home to the campus apartment which became a little second home for her. "I asked my doctor 'what can I develop right quick so I can get a handicapped parking sticker?' she jestfully quipped. "It wasn't long before I had my handicap sticker. I also bought a Tiger tag for the Fort Hays University Tigers. I'm proud to have that tag on my car." Being within a few months of 100 years of age Nola was still taking classes, living in her campus apartment, and driving her car.

Nola has always had a special interest in learning about history. She explained her interest this way: "History has always been of special interest to me and that is primarily what I have been enrolled in during my time at FHSU. God created the earth and then he populated it. History tells me what that population did with it during their time on earth, and that interests me," she said. "I have mainly focused on classes on American history, the Civil War, political issues, global environmental topics and I also studied Russian history." One of her history professors has said that he wishes that his younger students had the drive to excel that Nola exhibits. In class Nola often shared her personal memories of events being studied which made it more interesting and understandable to her classmates. She commented, "I feel like I have really made an impression on them with my stories. I don't think they will forget the things I shared with them... I remember when the Berlin Wall was torn down and the days before the

Soviet Union was formed in 1917 and when I was six years old and my father had to go register for the draft in World War I."

Nola's interest in history has blossomed into an interest in family genealogy and a desire for foreign travel. She has traveled to England, where her family came from, and has also visited France, Austria, Jordan, and Egypt. She went to Bad Sodden, Germany to do research on family ancestors. She has especially enjoyed Israel and has been there six or seven times.

As Nola has aged, she has also kept up with new technology. She was one of the first people in Hodgeman County to own and use a computer. She uses it daily to keep in touch with family and friends in the states and overseas. She is also a very active member of the Southwest Kansas Library Board and takes part in various community activities. She still uses her skills to assist with keeping the family farm records.

Regarding her longevity Nola commented, "I never think of my age, we don't die at a certain age, and if people didn't know they were getting to a certain age, I think they would be better off. Just because they reach the age where their mother or father died doesn't mean they will too. I like to celebrate birthdays, but age doesn't determine what you can accomplish and it isn't a reason you can do something. My advice is to just ignore your age." She is hopeful that her story of her accomplishments will encourage other senior adults. She continued, "If I can be an inspiration to people and encourage them to not just sit on the couch and watch television; but to get out and do something, it gives me a good feeling. In fact, it really appeals to me a lot," she added.

If you would meet Nola you would not think that she is 100 years old. She is a very pleasant white-haired lady with a complexion of a lady at least 20 years younger. Her energy level, dexterity, handwriting and various abilities are all very admirably those of a much younger lady.

We may wonder what it is that contributes to the alertness and energy level of this 103 year old lady. It doesn't appear to be longevity genes as she has no ancestral history of longevity. She indicates that during her lifetime she has eaten a fairly well balanced diet consisting of whole grains, many raw fruits and vegetables, seeds and nuts, meat (including red meat), dairy, and limited sweets. As she has lived on a farm during her lifetime, much of her food has been home grown, which is most healthy.

We note that she has always abstained from the use of alcohol and tobacco products. Such clean living is a definite plus.

Nola is a Christian of the Baptist faith. She faithfully attends her church, reads her Bible frequently, and observes regular prayer times which provide fellowship with her Lord. This also is a definite plus.

During her lifetime, she has been somewhat overweight but has brought her body mass into the normal range which she now maintains. This also is a plus. Her health is generally good which indicates a healthy immune system. She had breast cancer in 1983, but she was able to overcome it with surgery. Being able to snap back from her bout with cancer also indicates a healthy immune system.

Another big plus for Nola is that she is blessed with a large, very loving family and many friends. She is a very loving, caring person that has endeared herself to many people.

Finally, we observe that she keeps herself going both mentally and physically. She focuses on healthy attitudes and an upbeat outlook on life. She gets physical exercise by gardening and taking a daily 15 minute walk. Altogether, the pluses outweigh any deficiencies in her lifestyle. Her advice to others desiring to live a good, long life is to do all things in moderation but to abstain totally from alcohol and tobacco. We can expect that she may very well live to be a super-centenarian. She truly is a lady to be emulated.

Acknowledgement and appreciation are expressed to Charlene Watson, freelance writer and the Kansas Senior Times for their valuable contribution and permission for this biography.

> *The silver-haired head is a crown of glory, if it is found in the way of righteousness. Proverbs 16:31*

* * * * *

Ivis Meitler:

It is amazing that this accomplished musician actually was self- taught and went on to become a recording artist at 100 years of age. Ivis Meitler was born Ivis Peck on September 20, 1910 at Sylvan Grove, Kansas as the second of ten children in a family that had to struggle to get by. Her father did his best as a "jack-of–all-trades". Ivis said, "My dad was a locksmith, shoe cobbler, barber – he was everything. He had to be with ten kids."

While attending church, Ivis heard the old pump organ but fell in love with the piano. With the poor financial situation of her family, there was no money available for piano lessons, but that didn't hold Ivis back. Having a good ear for music, she was able to teach herself to play. She said, "I played by ear. If I could hear it, I could play it. I learned to play 'Twinkle, Twinkle Little Star' on the white keys and 'Peter, Peter Pumpkin Eater' on the black keys." As she continued to practice she became more proficient on the keyboard. Thus, driven by desire and with aptitude she was able to succeed. She played for Sunday School services at age 11 and at 14 she played for the evening church services at Rosette Evangelical Church. In high school she played for a dance band. Her brother and his friend were also members of the band. They played for various community events. For each event Ivis received $5.00 pay which went to her father to help with family expenses. She took pride that at 100 years of age she was still on the payroll playing for evening services at Trinity Lutheran Church.

Ivis graduated from Sylvan Grove High School and went on to attend a teacher's college in Hays, Kansas. With a desire to get an office job, she moved to Salina, Kansas in 1937 to attend Brown Mackie College. Only a year later she married Oscar Meitler, who was also a Sylvan Grove native. Their only child, Sherry, was born later that year.

Ivis has had several occupations. She taught in rural schools in Lincoln County, worked at a drug store and at an oil company, but perhaps her most pleasurable occupation was owning and operating a dance studio for nearly 29 years. "I learned to dance with my daughter," Ivis said. "I helped her practice, and it came easy with me."

In December 2010, she took her favorite position at the piano at Presbyterian Manor in Salina, Kansas for a two hour recording session. For her first recording, titled "The Second Century", she played some of her favorite tunes, including "St. Louis Blues", "The Entertainer", "Maple Leaf Rag", "Stardust", "Tea for Two" and "Red Wing".

This indefatigable lady, after only a short break, went on to do a second recording of her favorite Christmas tunes. This recording, titled

"My 100 Christmases", contains her interpretations of "Joy to the World", "It Came Upon a Midnight Clear", "O Come All Ye Faithful", "O Holy Night", "Silent Night", and "Jingle Bell Rock" During her recording events she played the songs entirely from memory.

Ivis loved nothing more than playing the piano and sharing her music with others. Every day about noon she went to the dining hall at Presbyterian Manor to entertain her fellow residents with her favorite renditions including "Tea For Two", "Stardust", and "Maple Leaf Rag". She played for about 20 minutes before joining her friends for lunch. She also played for chapel services, birthdays, and other manor events.

Ivis actually made her first recording about 13 years previous to the two recordings she made in December. On that occasion, she was requested to make a recording to be sold in support of her church's building campaign. She designated the funds derived from her later recordings to benefit the youth program at Trinity Lutheran Church, which she faithfully attended.

This lady was a glowing example of Elizabeth Arden's statement, "You're as old as you feel." Claiming she didn't require much sleep, she was up and going every morning at 6:00. She was always looking for things to do to assist the staff and fellow residents. She helped at the front reception desk at the manor, attended exercise classes, and played in four bridge groups in Salina. She also volunteered at her church, playing piano for the Sunday evening services and coordinating the Women's Bible Study Group. A fellow church member, Daran Neuschafer, described her as "a gracious lady who loved the kids at church and made sure to attend all of the youth services."

Everyone who knew her wondered at the energy that Ivis displayed Gayle Doll, director of the Kansas State University Center on Aging in Manahattan, Kansas, claims that only about 30 percent of longevity is due to genetics, while the other 70 percent is due to lifestyle. Doll says that there are two vital lifestyle factors that allow centenarians to live so long with physical and mental health. One is personality: "Ivis believed she still had things to do with her life," Doll said.

The other factor, Doll stated, is mindset. "In the past we thought that once we turned 100, we wouldn't be able to do anything. Now that mindset is changing. We know that people 100 and older can continue to contribute; that they still can remain active and healthy for a long time. Ivis thought of herself as younger, so she acted and felt younger."

Ivis had her share of tragedy in her life, but she took it in stride. Her husband died in 1987, and her daughter died at age 54 only a few years later in 1993. Ivis was 86 when she moved into Presbyterian Manor. She lived in independent living and did all of her own housework. Her pastor, Rev. Robert Schandel said, "Through her involvement and enthusiasm, she's been a real gift from God. She's had her difficulties in life but had a strong faith and was always looking for opportunities for ministry. Not everyone has had the health and energy she was given, so she always was looking to do something for others."

At 100 years of age Ivis stated that she didn't know why she had lived so long. She was convinced that it's important to live with a good attitude, to stay positive and not to grumble about things you have no control over. "You always have to look on the bright side, and keep busy, that's the main thing," she said, "I know I do too many things, but I don't want to give up anything either. It's too much fun doing everything."

Ivis departed this life at the age of 103 on August 27, 2014.

Appreciation is extended to the Salina (Kansas) Journal, Sharon Montague, Deputy Editor and reporter Gary Demuth for permission to use excerpts from their original articles published January 16, 2011 and February 3, 2011.

> **NOTE**: While visiting at Maples Mill, Illinois in the late 1980's, while at the Church of the Nazarene, this author met a lady, Gladys Wilcoxen, who was an excellent pianist and could also play the organ. I was told that she was nearly 100 years old and had difficulty reading music due to failing vision but could play any hymn from memory when the hymn title was announced. I later learned that Gladys lived to be 98 years old and died about 1989. A relative, Lois Mellert Smith Wilcoxen, whom I also met, lived to be 102 at her death in about 2009. Other Mellert family members also enjoyed longevity. Maples Mill is a strictly rural community where the church is the only

prominent building and the people live simply and are occupied by farming. They raise much of their food in gardens and preserve food for winter use.

* * * * *

Frank Woodruff Buckles:

This man, born February 1, 1901, survived to be the last living military veteran of World War I. His life spanned the twentieth century, which took us from the horse and buggy through World Wars I & II and succeeding wars to the use of plastics, television, and computers and into the space age. Frank died on February 27, 2011 at 110 years of age. The following is his story, written mostly in his own words, which was published as a part of his obituary.

The Beginning

"I was born on my father's farm north of Bethany in Harrison County Missouri on February 1, 1901. My father retired in 1905 and bought property in the small town of Coffey, where I started school. In 1910 he bought a farm in Vernon County near Walker, Missouri where we enjoyed country living. In December 1916, we moved to Dewey County, Oklahoma, near Oakwood. I was 15 at the time, and I accompanied a boxcar load of draft horses and equipment to the farm. I knew that my father was planning to arrange for a man to take the horses to Oklahoma. He would be paid $20 and transportation back to Missouri. I asked my father if I could do the job and he agreed. My parents came later by automobile. In the charming little frontier town of Oakwood, population 300, I worked at the bank, lived at the hotel, and went to high school. On 6 April 1917, the United States entered the Great War and patriotic posters appeared in the post offices."

Enlistment

"When summer vacation came I was invited to the Kansas State Fair in Wichita. While there I went to the Marine Corps recruiting office to enlist. I said that I was 18, but the understanding sergeant said that I was too young; I had to be 21. I went to Lamed, Kansas, to visit my father's mother who was living with my aunt and uncle who owned the bank in Larned. A week later I returned to Wichita and went to the Marine Corps recruiting station. This time I stated that I was 21. The same sergeant gave me a physical examination, but kindly told me that I was just not heavy enough. I tried the navy and passed the tests, but they were perhaps suspicious of my age and told me that I was flat-footed. I decided to try elsewhere, so I went to Oklahoma City. There I had no luck with either the Marines or the Navy. Then I tried the Army, but was asked for a birth certificate. I told them that public records were not made of births in Missouri at the time I was born, and the record would be in the family Bible. They accepted this and enlisted me in the Army on 14 August 1917. Thirteen of us were accepted at the recruiting station and given rail tickets to Fort Logan, Colorado, where those who were accepted were sworn into the regular U.S. Army. My serial number was 15577. In choosing the branch of the Army in which to serve, the old sergeant advised that the ambulance service was the quickest way to get to France because the French were begging for ambulance services. I followed his advice and was sent to Fort Riley, Kansas for training and trench casualty retrieval and ambulance operations."

The Great War

"The unit that I went overseas with was called the First Fort Riley Casual Detachment, which consisted of 102 men. The ranking officer was a sergeant. I have a photo of this unit taken at Fort Riley. We sailed from Hoboken, New Jersey, via Halifax Nova Scotia in December 1917, aboard the HMS Carpathia; the vessel famous for the rescue of the White Star Liner, Titantic, on 15 April 1912. Some of the officers and crew who made the rescue were aboard the Carpathia and were not adverse to describing the rescue. We docked in Glascow, Scotland and our unit traveled on to Winchester, England to await cross-channel shipment to France. A unit of the 6th Marines was operating Camp Hospital No. 35 near Winchester. Our unit was forced to replace the Marines who were sent on to France. While in England I drove a Ford ambulance, a motorcycle with a side-car and a Ford car for visiting dignitaries. Others walked. After some weeks in England, I requested a meeting with the commanding officer of the area, Colonel Jones of the 6th Cavalry. I asked to be sent to France and he explained that, he too, wanted to go to France but had to stay where he was ordered. I finally got an assignment to escort an officer to France who had been left behind by his original unit. In France I had various assignments and was at several locations. After Armistice Day I was assigned to a prisoner-of-war escort company to return prisoners back to Germany. After two years with the AEF (American Expeditionary Force), I returned home on the USS Pocahontas in January 1920. I was paid $143.90, including a $60 bonus."

Returning Home

I went to visit my parents, then decided to get a quick education in shorthand and typing at a business school in Oklahoma City. After four months of school I got a job at the post office, working 4:00 p.m. to midnight. I was paid 60 cents an hour. In one month I had enough money to take the train to Toronto, Ontario, Canada, where I got a job in the freight soliciting office of the White

Star Line Steamship Company. I also had a night job with the Great Northwest Telegraph Company. During the winter of 1921, I went to New York and got a job in the bond department of the prestigious Bankers Trust Company at 5th Avenue and 42nd Street. I used as reference the Oakwood, Oklahoma bank where I had worked at age 15. The steamship business had more appeal for me, but first I had to have some experience at sea. I got my first sea job with the old Munson Line as assistant purser of the ship, Western World, bound for Buenos Aires. I spent several years with the Grace Line, in both cargo and passenger ships on the west coast of South America, where an intimate knowledge of the countries and the language was required. World War II – In 1940, I accepted an assignment to expedite the movement of cargoes for the American President Lines in Manila. Unfortunately for me, my stay was extended by the Japanese invasion of the Philippines in 1941. I spent three –and-a-half years in Japanese prison camps at Santo Tomas and Los Banos. We were rescued by the 11th Airbourne Division on 23 Feburary 1945.

Home Again

"Life in San Francisco was pleasant after World War II. On 14 September 1946 I married Audrey Mayo of Pleasanton, California. She was born on a ranch and my people were landowners and farmers for generations. So, we decided it was time to give-up foreign assignments and come back to the land. We came to Gap View Farm, near Charles Town, West Virginia, in January 1954 to reside in the area where my forefather, Robert Buckles, his wife and 15 other families settled in 1732."

Frank Buckles continued to work on his farm, and up until the age of 103 still drove his tractor. His wife, Audrey, to whom he was married for over 50 years, passed away in 1999. Frank's daughter, Susannah, and her family lived with him on his farm near Charles Town, West Virginia and provided care for him until his death at the age of 110 years. His final services were held at Zion Episcopal Church in Charles Town on March 16, 2011.

George Will, writing for the Washington Post in May of 2008, mentioned that Frank Buckles was at that time still in good health, had an agile mind and spoke fluently. At 107 years of age, his eyes were still sharp enough for him to be a keen reader, and his voice was still deep and strong. As a memento, he still had the small tin cup from which he ate his meals during his Japanese imprisonment. His conservative bent is disclosed as he revealed Ronald Reagan as the favorite president of his lifetime.

Buckles served as the Honorary Chairman of the World War I Memorial Foundation which campaigned to have the District of Columbia War Memorial renamed as the National World War I Memorial. During this time, he had a meeting with President George W. Bush. Buckles was a member of several organizations, including the Masonic Lodge, Shriners, the Sons of Confederate Veterans, and the Sons of the American Revolution which is somewhat revealing of his heritage. At the close of World War I, he was awarded the World War I Victory Medal and the Army of Occupation of Germany Medal. He also was awarded the French Legion of Honor Medal. He was known to be a man who revered God in his life.

Life on his 330 acre farm was good for Frank Buckles. Here he lived a quiet peaceful life with his family. He ate a reasonable diet and enjoyed a glass of wine and a good cigar or his pipe after meals. He got as much fresh air and sunshine as possible. As he had a heart problem, he took some medications and specific vitamins that were helpful to him and used supplements such as fish oil and CoQ10. He had a special interest in longevity and always believed, as an aunt had told him when he was young, that he would live a long life. He seems to have had the genes for longevity as his father, two sisters, and some of his aunts, uncles, and cousins lived to 90 -100 years of age. Frank's advice for living a good long life was, "Relax; practice moderation in all things; keep moving (exercise daily); drink water, breathe fresh air and get lots of sunshine." Through all of the tribulations of his life this stalwart man continued on being a patriotic citizen, a good parent and a good neighbor in his community.

Appreciation is extended to Frank Buckles daughter, Susannah Flanagan, for granting permission to use his obituary and for supplementary information provided.

* * * * *

In this biographical section we have briefly described the lives and to some extent the lifestyles of several admirable Americans, some of whom are still living and some of whom have recently died. Although the depiction has been brief we can identify characteristics which make them admirable and which have contributed to their longevity.

> *"Measure not life by the hopes and enjoyments of this world, but by the preparation it makes for another; looking forward to what you shall be rather than backward to what you have been. He is not dead who departs from life with a high and noble fame; but he is dead, even while living, whose brow is branded with infamy"*   *– Tieck*

> *"He lives long that lives well; and time misspent is not lived but lost. God is better than His promise if he takes from him a long lease, and gives a freehold of a better value."*   *Fuller*

> *"I think the only reason you should retire is if you can find something you enjoy more than what you're doing now."*
>   *George Burns*

> *"We are happier in many ways when we are old than when we were young. The young sow wild oats. The old grow sage."*
>   *Sir Winston Churchill*

Chapter Three
What We Have Learned About Longevity

As we have studied the people of various cultures, we have learned that no one thing is responsible for longevity but that longevity depends upon a person's entire lifestyle. Here are some of the things observed that are important to reach your goal. These are not ranked in order of importance; they are all important and must be in concert to balance a harmonious longevity lifestyle wherein one can live long and live well.

1. **Genetics:** With the possible exception of Ovadda, the study of the world's cultures has not revealed that inherited genes play an overwhelming role in longevity. The average effect of genes is about 35%.

2. **Environment:** One of the areas we have studied is a very high mountain valley, three others are islands, and Loma Linda is located in a metropolis. It would seem that all except Loma Linda have good air quality. The people in the mountains and islands spend much time outdoors where they get fresh air. The people in Hunza have very good quality water. Although we have no specific information, the people living in island communities likely also have good water as some are mountainous. Only in Loma Linda is their quality of life threatened by poor air and water quality. In Loma Linda, they live a much different lifestyle, being indoors most of the time when their air quality is poorest.

Their water is treated to make it acceptable. Living in a place with good air and water quality is definitely preferable.

3. **Diet:** Although the diets of these peoples vary in some respects, they are all largely vegetarian with some exceptions. Although the Okinawans eat pork, they boil it to eliminate the fat. The Ovoddans eat some meat fairly regularly. None have beef as a dietary item. Some eat fish. The Seventh-Day Adventists shun eating any meat. The Mediterranean people typically use a lot of olive oil and include wine as a beverage. The SDA do not use any alcoholic beverages, and they don't use tobacco products. However, the diets of all were predominately whole grain bread, fruits, vegetables, whole grains, beans, and legumes. All except the Hunzas use a little low fat dairy, especially cheese and yogurt. Some drink goat milk.

4. **Mental attitude:** All of these people display a very positive mental attitude toward life and their livelihood. They look forward to every day and go about their tasks with a positive state of mind. They are self-disciplined to live right.

5. **Family and social life:** Family ties are valued, respected, and very strong. The people in all of these groups gather for family events and also for community festivals. They are very sociable with friends as they go about their daily activities.

6. **Stress and rest:** Life for all of these people is mostly low key. All get adequate rest. Some take naps, and the SDA are very adamant about strictly observing Saturday as their day of rest.

7. **Spiritual life:** The Hunzas are Muslim; the Okinawans are mostly Buddhists, with some being Christians; the Mediterranean people are Roman Catholic Christians and the SDA are Protestant Christians. All take their faith as a very serious part of their life and gain deep spiritual strength from their manner of worshipping God.

8. **Exercise:** Physical activity is very much a part of the daily routine for all of the cultures we have studied. The lone exception is the Seventh-Day Adventists who work at various occupations in the city. Some living in apartments or condominiums don't even do yard work or gardening. However, these people are encouraged to find ways to get daily exercise if only walking.

The Outlook for Longevity in the United States

The question on everyone's mind is, "what are my chances?" By now you should have a good idea about what it takes to live long and live well. Since longevity has been increasing in the United States and continues to increase at an accelerated rate for those who have the right lifestyle, your chances are very good. Even if you are overweight or have been a smoker you can still extend your lifespan if you start making the right choices now to get there.

A doctor friend once told me that "it is all in the genes." I disagreed then and am now even more firmly convinced because of what I have studied and observed. The evidence indicates that the genetic effect accounts for 20 to 50 percent of one's longevity. The average is 30 percent. That genetic rate would not likely take a person much beyond normal life expectancy. So if you desire to be a centenarian, you must do the right things to extend your life beyond the norm. Our studies demonstrate that those who do the right things can beat the odds. Even those at Loma Linda, who must contend with some poor environmental qualities, manage to excel in longevity at an outstanding rate. Furthermore, many who do not become centenarians still live beyond the norm.

Belle Shaw, who was a family friend, had a brother who lived actively beyond 100 years, but she died in her eighties. Howbeit, he was slender, while she was obese, which was a negative for her. The father of a doctor friend lived to be 102, but the doctor, being well educated on health matters, but was overweight, died in his eighties. Charles and Fern Scrivner, who have lived a good lifestyle, were still going at 101 and 94 years respectively. Both have outlived siblings. Of course, this sampling is much too small to be conclusive; however, it is a good indication that genetics is not the determining factor. Furthermore, if genetics were the determining factor, there would not be so many who die before reaching their normal life expectancy.

In the United States today, there are approximately 80,000 centenarians. You have a 1 in 80 chance of becoming a centenarian. So, if you are in a room with 79 other people, one of you has a good chance of becoming a centenarian IF you live the right lifestyle. Beyond that, at this writing, there are known to be 50 supercentenarians (those who live to 110 years and beyond) in the world, 15 of which are in the United States. Only three of the world's supercentenarians are men, and only one of these is in the United States. There are two possible explanations for the low number of male centenarians. Men generally labor harder and experience more physical stress, and men tend to be less spiritual than women. The oldest living women in the U.S at this writing are all Caucasians. Of these, the oldest are Eunice Sanborn (114, Texas) and Bessie Cooper (114, Georgia). The oldest living white man in the U.S. is Walter Bruening (also 114 years) who resides in Montana.

The oldest living African-American in the United States was **Mississippi Winn,** who died on January 28, 2011 at the age of 113 years. Winn, whose nickname was "Sweetie", was the daughter of slave parents. She was residing in a Shreveport, Lousiana nursing home at the time of her death. She had lived on her own until she was 103 years old and was in good health until just a few months before she died.

Winn was never married and had worked as a domestic. She was one of 15 children, eight of whom lived to adulthood. She had a brother who lived to be 95 and a sister who lived to be 100 years old. She enjoyed an abiding spiritual life. Her pastor commented that, "Her Church family and friends all loved and cherished her."

The Gerontology Research Group, which keeps records on and studies the statistics of centenarians, has projected that the number of centenarians in the United States will increase exponentially to 214,000 by 2020, to 324,000 by 2030, to 447,000 by 2040, and to a whopping 834,000 by 2050. If you aspire to be a centenarian, your chances are good, so go for it and do all the right things.

Chapter Four
The Physiology of Longevity

When an elderly person dies with no apparent reason, a doctor may say that the death was caused by "old age". This causes one to wonder what contributes to old age causing a person to die. As medical science has studied the human body, there is much that has been learned and there is much still being studied by a relatively new branch of medicine called Anti-Aging Medicine.

The human body is composed of a collection of interacting systems, each of which has its own combination of functions and purposes. These systems are 1) Nervous, 2) Musculosketal, 3) Circulatory, 4) Respiratory, 5) Gastrointestinal, 6) Integumentary (skin covering), 7) Urinary, 8) Reproductive, 9) Immune, and 10) Endrocrine (glands). Each of these systems supports in some manner all of the other systems so that the body can function in concert harmoniously as a whole.

The body is composed of as many as 100 trillion various cells. The health and replicative ability of the cell structure determines the longevity of the individual because the cell is the basic functional unit of life. Most cells are minute, but they can reach from the toe to the brain stem. Each cell is enclosed in a plasma membrane that separates it from its surroundings. Within each cell there are several little organs (organelles) that have various functions.

The **nucleus** is the most conspicuous organelle. It houses the cell's **chromosomes,** which contain almost all of the DNA. Tucked away inside the DNA of the genes are the instructions for how to construct a unique individual. At the end of each chromosome there are **telomeres,** which protect the chromosome from deterioration. These telomeres suffer from wear with each replication (cloning) to create new cells. This damage makes the telomere a little shorter. When the telomere reaches a critically short length, the cell enters "replicative senescence" becoming no longer able to divide and is therefore dysfunctional and excretes enzymes and proteins that are toxic to adjoining cells. This inability to replicate telomeres shortens an individual's life span.

Growth or healing in the body is by this process of cell division which involves a single mother cell that divides into two daughter cells. The two primary building blocks of cells are protein (about 60%) and fat (about 40%). The process of cell division requires certain proteins to complete the process. The enzyme **telomerase** can replace short bits of the telomeres which are otherwise shortened when a cell divides, thus rejuvenating the life of the cell. The gene that codes for this enzyme exists in every one of our cells; however, in normal adult cells it is regulated in such manner that it is rendered ineffective to prevent telomere erosion. NOTE: The telomerase is 'switched on' in cancer cells causing them to reproduce inordinately to become "immortal' and form tumors.

Telomere shortening can be controlled naturally by diet and exercise up to a point. Scientists have been searching for the real solution to the problem by finding ways to safely promote telomerase activation. Telomerase activation in aged or chronically stressed normal cells has been shown to slow or reverse telomere shortening, increase replicative capacity, and restore or improve cellular function. Thus telomerase re-regulates the clock that controls the life span of the dividing cells.

In 2001, scientists at Geron, a biotech company, discovered TA-65, a proprietary, single molecule purified from Astragalus Botanical Roots that causes telomerase activation. This discovery gives promise of being a virtual "Fountain of Youth". Where there is a concern consumption of PQQ is recommended for mitochondrial health. The manufacturer says that, "while it will not cure any age-related disease, it will enhance the user's own cellular function and the amazing thing about telomerase activation therapy is that users report skin pores become smaller almost overnight, wrinkles disappear, greater skin metabolic ability to repair or correct cellular, organal, hormonal or skin-related problems. Each individual in our tests has shown different results as the age-related symptoms themselves differ from person-to-person."

Regarding this discovery the Journal of the American Medical Association has said (according to an online advertisement),

> "This advance not only suggests that telomeres are the central timing mechanism for cellular aging, but also demonstrates that such a mechanism can be reset, extending the replicative life span of such cells and resulting in markers of gene expression typical of "younger" (i.e., early passage) cells without the hallmarks of malignant transformation. It is now possible to explore the fundamental cellular mechanisms underlying human aging, clarifying the role played by replicative senescence."

Mitochondria are other organelles that are important in the aging process. These are within the cells in various numbers, shapes, and sizes. They are also self-replicating organelles. They are essentially important because they generate energy to power the cell.

The primary task of mitochondria is to create adenosine triphosphate (ATP). This is done in various energy cycles that involve nutrients such as Acetyl-L-Carnitine, CoQ10, NADH, and other nutrients, including some B vitamins.

ATP is the essential life-giving chemical because every function of every body part is generated from it. As the cell can store only a very little ATP, a constant supply must be produced. Therefore the mitochondria must be healthy and efficient so that they can produce the constant supply needed for repair and regenerative processes. Body organs cannot borrow energy from each other, so the efficiency of the mitochondria of each organ is essential to prevent it from failing and perhaps dying.

It can be seen that enhancement and protection of the health of mitochondria is essential to prevent or slow the aging process. When the mitochondria are damaged by trauma or aging pathologies, they are released from dying tissue and may be recognized as foreign bacteria, sometimes triggering an acute or chronic inflammatory response. The loss of healthy, functional mitochondria can lead to death of the individual.

Life Extension Magazine has reported on some recent research regarding mitochondria health and the discovery of a substance, called PQQ *(pyrroloquinoline quinine)*, that can prevent mitochondrial decay as its chemical structure enables it to withstand extreme oxidation. "When combined with CoQ10, research shows that just 20 mg per day of PQQ can significantly preserve and enhance memory, attention and cognition in aging humans." But the most exciting revelation on PQQ emerged in early 2010, when researchers found that it not only protected mitochondria from oxidative damage - it also stimulated growth of new mitochondria!."[4]

This discovery is very important for the prevention of brain aging. "It has been shown to optimize the function of the entire central nervous system" (p.6). This is valuable to those with early onset of Parkinson's or Alzheimer's, stroke victims and those who need cardiovascular biogenesis. It is available without prescription as it is an alternative treatment.

Noticeably aging, wrinkled skin is indicative of cell degeneration, whereas a smooth, clear skin complexion with good resilience indicates healthy cellular structure. Scientists at the Cellular Life Research Center at St. Petersburg, Florida have made a remarkable discovery regarding cellular health. Body cells produce certain proteins, each of which is responsible for a certain function. When these proteins become damaged, residues called Abnormal Aspartyls are formed. The residue of Abnormal Aspartyls in cells causes a deficiency in cellular structure which disturbs the biological function of the proteins. This causes aging. Unless stopped these Abnormal Aspartyls can affect the health of body cells, including those in the joints, the heart, the pancreas, the liver, and the brain. Scientists have discovered that to stop this degenerative process our bodies must produce an adequate supply of an enzyme called PIMT. They have successfully produced it in a 100% natural product called PIMT4Life. This product was released to the medical community in late 2009, and it was voted to be the best scientific breakthrough of 2010. It was released to the public in 2011. The scientists at the center believe that this product has the anti-aging ability to prevent many diseases and extend life to 100 or possibly even 150 years. The results are already being seen in the skin, nails, muscular strength, and sensory functions of participating individuals.[5]

The Free Radical Theory of Aging, developed by Denham Harman,

M.D. at the University of Nebraska in 1956, has become very popularly accepted. Free radicals are created in the process of oxidation within our cells. The medical dictionary defines oxidation as, "Any chemical reaction in which a material gives up electrons, as when the material combines with oxygen. Burning is an example of rapid oxidation; rusting is an example of slow oxidation."

When oxidation occurs a free radical forms that can react with other substances in the body. Cells are composed of many different kinds of molecules. Molecules consist of atoms joined by chemical bonds. When weak bonds split, free radicals are formed. These free radicals are very unstable and attack other compounds trying to find a place of stability. Usually a free radical attacks the nearest stable molecule to attempt to steal its electron. When this occurs and the stable molecule loses its electron, that electron then becomes a free radical. Thereby, a chain reaction is created that can result in serious disruption of a living cell. Because oxygen is so reactive, it can initiate this process.

Antioxidants are the peacemakers that neutralize free radicals by donating one of their own electrons, thus ending the skirmish. They go on patrol, helping to prevent the weakening of cells that could lead to cellular damage, disease, and death. Antioxidants are numerous and include vitamins C, D, and E and resveratrol. The most effective antioxidant ever found is a form of lipoic acid. As antioxidants seem to be selective to various free radicals, a selection of varying antioxidants may be most effective in controlling free radicals.

An individual's life, processes of eating, drinking, and breathing requires energy created by the mitochondria, so free radicals are naturally formed. The production of free radicals is accelerated when the individual's lifestyle includes the use of tobacco, alcohol, and other drugs or is otherwise stressed. When a substantial number of an individual's cells become weakened and are unable to replicate themselves, that is when the individual dies of old age.

The Role of Hormones

Have you ever wondered how it is that our bodies undergo changes as we grow older? In your day-to-day life you may not be doing anything so different. You may be eating good meals, getting lots of sleep, and getting regular physical check-ups from your doctor, but, just as you saw changes in your strength and development during your teenage years, you are now seeing changes in the other direction. The answer is to be found in quiet natural processes involving your bodily hormones. As you were a teenager growing older, your hormone levels were increasing to fuel your development. When you were in your mid-twenties, your supply of hormones began to diminish. We are now going to look at what we can do about that to slow the aging process. It's not quite like stepping on the brake pedal in your car, but in some instances there are things we can do about it.

DHEA *(dehydroepiandrosterone):* The name is nearly impossible to pronounce, so it is most often simply called "DHEA". This is a steroid hormone that has been the subject of thousands of clinical studies, so we have much information concerning it. It is the most prevalent hormone produced by the adrenal glands. After being secreted, it circulates through the bloodstream as DHEA-sulfate (DHEA-S). It is then converted to other hormones as needed. These include important hormones like testosterone, estrogen, corticosterone and progesterone. It has been found to function differently in men, premenopausal women, and postmenopausal women.

This hormone is synthesized in the body, so dietary matters are not a consideration regarding the amount in the body. The level of DHEA may range as high as 700 in youth. Aging is not kind to our supply of DHEA. It is at its peak in youth at about the age of twenty-one years. From there, it decreases steadily until, at sixty, the supply is only about ten-to-fifteen percent and, by eighty years, the production is a mere five percent of what it was at its peak. This is sad because of its great importance to our bodily functions.

Fortunately the good news is that this hormone is available in a synthetic form in various dosages up to 100 mg. It is a good idea to occasionally obtain a blood test to determine the amount of DHEA circulating in the blood. This will give a knowledgeable point from which to determine the amount of supplementation needed. A desirable goal for adults would be to maintain a level no less than 250 with a goal of moving closer to 500. Supplementation of 100mg is not uncommon but rarely exceeds 200mg. Therapeutically larger doses have been taken but should be administered under doctor supervision. It is noted that DHEA appears to be safe even with high dosages.

DHEA is so active in bodily functions that it would be nearly impossible to overstate its importance. Researchers have found that it plays a very significant role in regulating the immune system. It increases the amount of estrogen in women and testosterone in men to more youthful levels; it decreases the tendency of blood platelets to stick together, reducing the incidence of heart attacks or strokes; it is anti-inflammatory; and weight lifters like it because it helps to boost endurance and build muscle mass.

This hormone can be very helpful in a weight loss program because it promotes fat burning and suppresses the appetite. It has the ability to improve the process of transforming food into energy instead of storing it as fat. Many have found that fat loss is accompanied with an increase in muscle mass. If being overweight is causing a person to have a blood sugar problem, this hormone will help to stabilize the sugar. In a diet such as the one we are suggesting, DHEA will be one key to achieving desired results.

One of the serious problems with aging is age-related diseases. We have noted that DHEA naturally decreases as people grow older. There is a direct correlation between this and the onset of these diseases. Appropriately supplementing the supply of DHEA can inhibit many diseases such as cardiovascular disease, cancer, lupus, osteoporosis, arthritis, and dementia and may even control the progress of these afflictions. It is also found to be helpful to manage age-related physiological changes such as menopause. It is indeed true that by maintaining a good level of DHEA an individual can extend her or his lifespan.

According to the Life Extension manual "Disease Prevention and Treatment"[6] researchers in Germany and Italy have found that there may be a definite benefit for postmenopausal women to take 50 mg of DHEA daily. As we have pointed out, DHEA is a precursor of estrogen and testosterone. The German study showed "decreased symptoms of depression and anxiety and increased libido". The Italian study concluded that "50 mg of DHEA taken for six months mimics the benefits of traditional hormone replacement therapy (HRT)." The study further indicated that the DHEA prevented a decrease in bone calcium and the onset of osteoporosis.

The Life Extension manual (pp.703-704) also reveals that DHEA provides some benefits for the skin. When applied topically to seriously burned areas, it saved the skin and blood vessels under the burned area. We do not yet know how this saves the skin but assume that anti-inflammatory action may be the reason for this.

DHEA also has skin-enhancing effects because it provokes the production of collagen and hyaluronic acid, both of which have proven benefits to the skin. Women who take DHEA orally have thicker skin, but the best results are derived from applying DHEA topically. These preparations also protect skin from daily wear and tear and from pollutants that could cause skin cancer.

When learning of all the benefits of DHEA, one may come to think of it as a *Fountain of Youth*. This is not the case as It does not reverse aging or promote immortality, but it definitely is worth taking by those who are middle-aged or older for the preservation benefits it provides.

Testosterone and estrogen are the dominant male and female hormones. It is what makes a male different from a female. It must be noted, however, that both men and women have testosterone and estrogen hormones. When they are young men have more testosterone and women have more estrogen. We are discussing them together because of the ways they affect both men and women.

Testosterone does many things besides defining masculinity. It helps to control bone density; it can control and reduce fat deposits and increase lean body mass; it affects the energy level of the body; it influences sexual ability, fertility, and erectile dysfunction; a lack of it can lead to high blood pressure and related heart problems. It also influences our mental ability, mood, our sense of well being, mental fatigue, anxiety level, and ability to focus and concentrate.

Not as much is known about testosterone in women, but we do know that it has some of the same functions that have been mentioned. We know that it has a vital role in ovarian health and that it influences libido and mood. Post-menopausal women are in danger of testosterone deficiency and need to be aware of its need for their well-being in this stage of life; however, it also affects younger women.

Testosterone is a steroid compound made from cholesterol. Considering its many functions, we can see that it has potent effects on the body. Adequate amounts of testosterone are necessary for longevity. The more testosterone a man has, the longer he lives. A lack of testosterone is referred to as "testosterone deficiency disease". Only in the past decade are doctors slowly beginning to recognize that testosterone deficiency greatly increases the chance of the onset of many diseases. The University of Washington has done research which shows a positive connection between low testosterone and increased mortality rates. Indeed testosterone deficiency can be fatal regardless of your sexual ability.

The 2009 Collector's Edition of Life Extension (Pp.95-100) published an article introducing the book "Testosterone for Life" by Abraham Morgentaler, M.D., Associate Clinical Professor at Harvard Medical School. In the book, Dr. Morgentaler points out the many fallacies that the medical profession has believed about testosterone deficiency and the seriousness of it.

Life Extension states, "Our position is that low testosterone contributes to the degenerative diseases of aging such as *chronic inflammation, neurologic decline, diabetes* and *atherosclerosis.*" The article also stated, "In our observations from the thousands of blood tests we perform each year for members… we found that men with <u>low</u> testosterone appear to be more likely to contract prostate cancer." [7]

Dr. Edward Lichten, M.D., F.A.C.S., has been in practice for over 30 years treating, researching, inventing and rediscovering ways to use bio-identical and natural therapies to treat his patients' diseases. In his *Textbook of Bio-Identical Hormones* he says, "One of the most important concepts that I have advanced is that high free sex hormone states correlate directly to health and that low free hormone states correlate with disease states. . . Testosterone is good for men and estrogen is good for women. The corollary is also true; too much of the wrong sex hormone and the wrong amount of SHBG will be found in an individual who is or will be at risk for diabetes and disease." [8]

The pituitary gland located at the base of the brain is the "command center" that secretes a hormone to send a message to the testicles (or ovaries) and adrenal glands to produce testosterone. Testosterone is another hormone that diminishes in the body after a man reaches middle-age (35-45 years). This decrease is caused due to the negative effect of estrogen in a man's body. Estrogen affects the production of a protein called sex hormone-binding globulin (SHBG). This SHBG tightly binds testosterone, making it inactive. Therefore there are two measures of testosterone in a man's body. One is bound testosterone, and the other is free testosterone. Together they are called total testosterone. The only active testosterone is free testosterone, and it is now being limited.

Dr. Lichten says, "Not only does estrogen compete with testosterone for penetration into the cell; it competes for production from the pituitary stimulating hormones"[9]

There is an old joke about which came first, the chicken or the egg. Similarly, scientists used to wonder which came first, abdominal fat or testosterone deficiency. It is known that fat does cause a drop in testosterone levels, but scientists now believe that the decrease in testosterone came first. With the decrease, men's breasts tend to enlarge and they get increasing amounts of belly fat. Now here is the thing that is supremely important for everyone to know. **It is impossible for a man to get rid of his enlarged breasts and big belly if his free testosterone level is too low.** No matter how you control your diet or how much you exercise, you will not be able to eliminate the fat. This may also be true for women. Keep in mind also that testosterone deficiency disease will seriously shorten your life.

The really bad news is that SHBG is an estrogen amplifier, so as the amount of testosterone gets lower the amount of bad estrogen in the form of estrodial increases appreciably and can create a severe testosterone/estrogen imbalance. When this happens the breasts and belly continue to enlarge; the man may experience heavy night sweats and his prostate may enlarge so much that his urine stream slows as the swollen prostate squeezes the ureter. It could become very difficult, or even impossible, to urinate. This blockage of urine flow may cause a urinary tract infection (UTI). So now we understand just how critical it is to maintain a good level of testosterone in the man's body.

If a woman does not have enough testosterone, she may be overweight, moody, and may not be energetic. She may have little libido, be unable to enjoy her relationship with her spouse, and be more susceptible to osteoporosis. Therefore she loses interest in sexual desires. Both men and women need to understand this phenomenon and if it occurs take steps to correct the condition. Women who have undergone the therapy suggested herein have been seen to lose weight and regain their more pleasing figure.

The *Life Extension* article cited states, "Building muscle mass and bone density while reducing abdominal fat are well-established improvements in body composition observed in response to testosterone therapy. *Testosterone for Life* relates recent data showing that testosterone not only helps to increase the strength and size of each muscle cell, but also influences nearby cells into becoming muscle cells."[10]

The first step in correcting testosterone deficiency is to have a doctor order blood testing for free testosterone, total testosterone, and estrodial, and with men should also request a PSA to check for the possibility of prostate cancer. There are various tests that are used but the important thing is that the free testosterone level should be within one-third of the upper level. Additionally, the doctor will need to make a clinical assessment considering all of the symptoms together with the test information. Even when the level may be said to be acceptable, testosterone replacement may be warranted due to the signs and symptoms.

The *Life Extension* article, previously indicated, gives suggestions concerning test levels. "We at *Life Extension* suggest that aging men maintain their *free testosterone* at a level of 20-25 pg/ml to more closely resemble that of a healthy 21 year old."

It used be thought that if prostate cancer is suspected testosterone replacement should not be done because this could make the cancer worse. Some doctors now believe that cancer is caused due to a lack of testosterone and that testosterone replacement is worth the risk as it may, in fact, prevent cancer from advancing. If a doctor discourages treatment, it is worth requesting a second or third opinion by the most competent doctors you can find. Some doctors just don't feel competent to deal with this.

Doctors treat testosterone deficiency with a series of injections. There is also a testosterone cream available by prescription which seems to be equally effective. Recently we have become aware of a non-prescription bio-identical homeopathic testosterone cream for men which is cost effective and reportedly provides good results.

There are also some natural herbal products that are helpful in treating this problem. The first is diindolymethane (DIM) which is derived from cruciferous vegetables of the cabbage family, like broccoli. It is an indole – a plant compound with healing properties. It has been found in study animals to prevent cancer. More recently it has been found to balance the sex hormones testosterone and estrogen.

DIM goes to the root of the problem because it stimulates more efficient estrogen metabolism by breaking down estrogen into its good metabolites. This is beneficial to menopausal women. Production of the "bad" metabolite (estradiol) is promoted by obesity and some environmental factors. The use of DIM by men results in a more desirable relationship of estrogen to testosterone by balancing the active bad estrogen in the male body. The good estrogen metabolites promote more free testosterone because it is removed from the testosterone binding proteins.

The production of more testosterone can be induced by taking a supplement called testofen. This product is derived from fenugreek. The producer, Gencor Pacific, has conducted some in-house studies which indicate that it:

"a. Stimulates natural androgen (testosterone) production by acting on the adrenals and pituitary gland and
b. Binds independently to testosterone receptor sites to stimulate androgenic/anabolic responses."

Practical experience seems to verify these findings but it would be good to have independent tests to further verify these results.

Dr. E. Barry Gordon of Brooklyn, New York has been a pioneer in discovering and treating testosterone deficiency disease. More information regarding his findings may be found in the resources section at the end of this book. Early-on, some doctors disputed his findings, but they are coming to be accepted more and more as he presents experiential evidence and others present findings that are in agreement.

Note: The information concerning hormones given herein is not intended to diagnose or cure any physical condition but is given for educational purposes only. In the plan of creation men and women were created such that various hormone levels in all individuals naturally decrease as human men and women age. Higher hormone levels are important for men and women during the early years of life for adequate growth and development and in married life for the spouses to express love and for procreation. This purpose diminishes as men and women age beyond their child-bearing years. However, we now know that adequate hormone levels are important to protect aging individuals from various diseases often referred to as diseases of old age. For health reasons it is important to maintain healthy hormone levels. The reader is warned that sexual activity outside of wedlock between one man and one woman can lead to serious sexually transmitted diseases. These diseases exist because immoral sexual activity violates the plan of creation and is considered to be sin against our Creator, Who is divinely recognized as God.

Human Growth Hormone (HGH) is a hormone that is produced by the pituitary gland. During our growing years, this hormone is responsible for controlling all of our growth processes so that they are always adequately progressing and under control. Like the production rates of other hormones, the production rate of HGH decreases in the pituitary until by the age of 70 years very little is found to be active in the bloodstream. This causes a condition that is called somatopause.

When an individual is in somatopause visible signs of aging that cause some emotional distress are visible. These may include wrinkled and sagging skin, balding, muscle loss, decreased energy, bone thinning, less manliness, and memory problems. The pituitary gland is still capable of producing HGH; however, there are factors that occur in the aging body that prevent this release of HGH into the bloodstream.

Over 50 years ago, while experimenting with various ingredients, a doctor discovered that Procaine apparently had an effect on the pituitary which stimulated the release of HGH into the bloodstream causing physical improvements resembling age reversal. Ingredients that cause this reaction are called secretagogues. With this discovery, the search was on to discover other possible secretagogues that would stimulate the release of HGH from the pituitary. Today, there are several products on the market whose manufacturers claim that they cause signs of age reversal. You will find some of these in the resource section in the back of this book.

The medical establishment is slow to recognize the claims made for these secretagogues regarding the slowing or, in some circumstances, the reversal, of aging. Many clinical trials have been done on a wide variety of aspects regarding the use of HGH with generally promising positive results. The doctors of Mayo Clinic acknowledge that injections of HGH can result positively in increased muscle mass and decreases in body fat but warn that there can also be side effects such as joint or muscle pain. Regarding the synthetic secretagogues they remain skeptical and call for more testing. So, as usual, the promoters of alternatives are ahead, leading the way with research and the production of HGH secretagogues.

Those who have used one of these secretagogues that have been on the market for over 30 years give very positive testimonials reporting outstanding results regarding their use of this product. They report greatly increased energy levels, fewer problems with arthritis, less pain from previous injuries, age spots disappearing, more youthful appearance, stronger nails, hair being thicker and gray diminishing to the previous color or very slowly graying, improved eyesight, better sleep, fewer asthma problems, stronger immune systems, less depression, a sense of well-being, and general improvement in their health.

Other users of HGH products report fat loss and muscle gain, increased libido, more satisfying sexual performance, improved skin elasticity, diminished wrinkling, lower blood pressure, and a greater sense of balance. Of course, the results vary with the product and the individual, so not all have the same results, but all do seem to find improvements.

Gary Null, PhD, the author of *Power Aging*, states, "Experts disagree on the benefits of supplementing with growth hormone. Some are excited about the anti-aging benefits seen in scientific studies. In these studies, senior citizens given growth hormone show an increase in lean muscle mass, a decrease in body fat, increased energy, stronger immune systems, sharper eyesight, and better mental acuity. Other experts, however, caution that more research into safe amounts is needed."[11]

There are four delivery systems for HGH products. The first of these is by injection. This must be prescribed and administered by a doctor. There are three downsides to this method. The injections may be painful, they must be repeated at intervals, and they are quite expensive. However, they are effective.

The second delivery system is to take the synthetic secretagogue in pill form. The downside of pills is that some of the ingredients are lost in the digestive process. However, they are available without a prescription and many users have found them to be effective. If the pill contains niacin, some users report some skin flushing as a side effect. There are several different products with differing secretagogues. They must be taken continuously but are generally cost effective.

Another means of boosting HGH is by consuming a powdered formula that is mixed with water. These are known to have niacin in the formula, which can give the user a very unpleasant niacin flush. This is a warm prickly feeling accompanied by the skin turning red from head to foot. When taken on an empty stomach, the concoction may cause this effect within five minutes of consumption, and the flush may last 30 minutes. One thing about the flushing is that it indicates that the ingredients are getting to every cell of the body. If an individual can adjust to and tolerate the flushing, which may vary in severity from day to day, this form is acceptable. If the individual is consuming other products containing niacin, the flushing will be more severe. Some users don't seem to have the problem with flushing. When considering this form of delivery, it is advisable to carefully check the ingredients.

The final delivery system is by using a spray product. This is simply sprayed into the mouth and held there under the tongue, as much as possible, until it is absorbed into the tissue of the mouth. This delivery system has been found to be effective as it gets into the bloodstream quickly without any loss by the digestive process. The cost of this product is not prohibitive. The producer of one of these currently offers a 90-day money back guarantee.

Thyroid Hormone is another hormone that can stand in the way of weight loss if it is underactive. This condition is called hypothyroidism. An overactive thyroid is called hyperthyroidism. Our consideration here is mainly of hypothyroidism, which is far more common than is usually recognized.

An individual with an underactive thyroid may notice cold hands and feet, cold intolerance, fatigue, muscular weakness, slow body movement, swollen eyelids, and/or ankles, dry skin and brittle nails, difficulty concentrating or remembering, nervousness, irritability, moodiness, depression and of course persistent weight gain with appropriate caloric intake and the concomitant inability to lose fat.

If an individual suspects a hypothyroid condition a further indication is one's basal temperature. This can be checked by keeping a thermometer on the bed stand for use upon awakening in the morning. Before getting out of bed place the thermometer under an armpit to check your temperature. Be sure to leave it there long enough. The body functions best with a temperature of 97.8 – 99.8 degrees. If the basal temperature is lower than this it is an indication of a possible problem that should be further checked by a doctor familiar with hormonal treatment.

Doctors use blood tests to check an individual's thyroxine (T4) and triodothyronine (T3). The thyroid stimulating hormone (TSH) should also be checked. The production of thyroid is another function that is stimulated by the pituitary gland, so we are further impressed with the importance of this little gland at the base of the brain. These tests are not always conclusive and should be considered along with a clinical examination which considers all of the symptoms.

A cold body does not function adequately. Therefore, when hypothyroidism exists, the body metabolism is too low for effective fat burning so the fat tends to accumulate mostly in the waist, abdomen, buttocks, and thighs but will eventually include the whole body if unchecked. The production of T3 is on an "as needed" basis, so if an individual is dieting the body may sense a need to conserve fuel; simply eating less in and of itself may not effectively treat obesity.

Hypothyroidism may be caused by a mineral or chemical deficiency. It has been found that a deficiency of iodine causes goiter and that is why iodine is typically added to salt. However, the amount of iodine added to salt, while sufficient to prevent goiter problems, may be insufficient to prevent hypothyroidism which hides under the surface contributing to health problems. Also if a dieting person curtails salt intake, the individual does not benefit from this source. Iodine is added to many multiple vitamin-mineral supplements, though, which can provide another source. An adequate supply of essential trace elements is a good reason for taking a quality vitamin-mineral supplement daily.

Eating or breathing of toxic substances might contribute to hypothyroidism. The fluoride and chlorine which are added to municipal drinking water could be the culprit. Coffee and beverages with caffeine could be contributors. Mercury is very hazardous and can be in the fillings in our teeth or ingested by eating fish. Inhaling the smoke of tobacco products or simply eating an improper diet could be problematic. Those who follow The Longevity Diet will eliminate many of these possible sources of thyroid problems.

Traditional doctors may treat an underactive thyroid with synthroid or Armour Thyroid which can be an effective treatment. However, such drugs do have side effects and interactions or reverse reactions which may resemble symptoms of hyperthyroidism, such as heat intolerance, headaches, or irritability. The drugs are known to possibly interact with many classes of medications. So, it may be best to first try to eliminate the possible causes that we can identify and proceed accordingly with treatment.

A more natural approach is to treat hypothyroidism with vitamins, minerals, and supplements as has already been suggested. Those that are important are vitamin A, vitamin B complex, vitamin B12, vitamins C, D3, E and coenzyme Q10 along with iodine, zinc, selenium, magnesium, molybdenum and manganese. A deficiency of tyrosine will lead to hypothyroidism, so if that is detected 1 gram per day would be adequate for adults. The amino acid L-tyrosine is also needed in conjunction with the foregoing for proper metabolism. A nutritional doctor will be helpful in determining this course of treatment.

Several hormones have been discussed here and all are equally important to support a healthy, well-functioning body. Aging occurs when our hormone levels decrease, therefore it is important for good health, optimal weight, and longevity to maintain all of the hormone levels appropriately. All of our hormones and body functions need to work harmoniously in concert to keep us going in peak condition. An example is that adequate DHEA is necessary for proper thyroid functioning. It appears that there is a connection between HGH and thyroid as those on HGH therapy experience a very notable increase in energy levels and weakness (lack of energy) is also a symptom of hypothyroidism. Remember that both HGH and TSH are stimulated from the pituitary so what stimulates one may also stimulate another. Blood testing is recommended to determine hormone levels and then use hormone replacement therapy using, inasmuch as possible, bio-identical hormones or other treatment that has been suggested herein with the guidance of an appropriate physician. The bottom-line on hormones is that older men and women who are hormone deficient are susceptible to disease and early death.

The Digestive System

To understand proper diet, nutrition and eating habits it is important to know some things about the human digestive system and the things that we put in it

The digestive system is made up of the digestive tract – a series of hollow organs joined in a long twisting tube from the mouth to the anus – and other organs that help the body break down and absorb food.

The organs that make up the digestive tract are the mouth, esophagus, stomach, small intestine, large intestine (also called the colon), rectum, and anus. Inside these hollow organs is a lining called the mucosa. In the mouth, stomach, and small intestine, the mucosa contains tiny glands that produce juices to help digest food. The digestive tract also contains a layer of smooth muscle that helps to break down food and move it along the tract.

Two solid digestive organs, the liver and the pancreas, produce digestive juices that reach the intestine through small tubes called ducts. The gallbladder stores the liver's digestive juices until they are needed in the intestine. Parts of the nervous and circulatory systems also play major roles in the digestive system.

Why is digestion important?

When you eat foods – such as bread, meat, and vegetables- they are not in a form the body can use as nourishment. Food and drink must be changed into smaller molecules of nutrients before they can be absorbed into the blood and carried to cells throughout the body. Digestion is the process by which food and drink are broken down into their smallest parts so the body can use them to build and nourish cells and to provide energy.

How is food digested?

Digestion involves mixing food with digestive juices, moving it through the digestive tract, and breaking down large molecules of food into smaller molecules. Digestion begins in the mouth, where food is mixed with enzymes when you chew and swallow, and is completed in the small intestine.

The movement of food through the system.

The large, hollow organs of the digestive tract contain a layer of muscle that enables their walls to move. The movement of organ walls can propel food and liquid through the system and can also mix the contents within each organ. Food moves from one organ to the next through muscle action called peristalsis. Peristalsis looks like an ocean wave traveling through the muscle. The muscle of the organ contracts to create a narrowing and then propels the narrowed portion slowly down the length of the organ. These waves of narrowing push the food and fluid in front of them through each hollow organ.

The first major muscle movement occurs when food or liquid is swallowed. Although you are able to start swallowing by choice, once the swallow begins, it becomes involuntary and proceeds under the control of the nerves.

Swallowed food is pushed into the esophagus, which connects the throat above with the stomach below. At the junction of the esophagus and stomach, there is a ringlike muscle, called the lower esophageal sphincter, closing the passage between the two organs. As food approaches the closed sphincter, the sphincter relaxes and allows the food to pass through to the stomach.

The stomach has three mechanical tasks. First, it stores the swallowed food and liquid. To do this, the muscle of the upper part of the stomach relaxes to accept large volumes of swallowed material. The second job is to mix up the food, liquid, and digestive juice produced by the stomach. The lower part of the stomach mixes these materials by its muscle action. The third task of the stomach is to empty its contents slowly into the small intestine. It takes approximately two hours after eating for the stomach to empty.

Several factors affect emptying of the stomach, including the kind of food and the degree of muscle action of the emptying stomach and the small intestine. Carbohydrates, for example, spend the least amount of time in the stomach, while protein stays in the stomach longer and fat the longest. As the food dissolves into the juices from the pancreas, liver, and intestine, the contents of the intestine are mixed and pushed forward to allow further digestion.

Finally, the digested nutrients are absorbed through the intestinal walls and transported throughout the body. The waste products of this process include undigested parts of the food, known as fiber, and older cells that have been shed from the mucosa. These materials are pushed into the colon, where they remain until the feces are expelled by a bowel movement.

Due to the importance of the intestines in transporting nutrients into the cells of the body, it is important to keep the intestines and colon cleansed so that they can function efficiently. Eating foods high in fiber and staying well hydrated is a natural way of cleansing but there are also products that are helpful in this regard.

Production of digestive juices

The digestive glands that act first are in the mouth—the salivary glands. Saliva produced by these glands contains an enzyme that begins to digest the starch from food into smaller molecules. An enzyme is a substance that speeds up chemical reactions in the body.

The next set of digestive glands is in the stomach lining. These glands produce stomach acid and an enzyme that digests protein. A thick mucus layer coats the mucosa and helps keep the acidic digestive juice from dissolving the tissue of the stomach itself. In most people, the stomach mucosa is able to resist the juice, although food and other tissues of the body cannot.

The process of digestion in the intestines is aided or hindered by bacteria in the intestines. Good bacteria aides digestion and promotes good health, while bad bacteria promotes unhealthy conditions. Taking antibiotics kills both the good and bad bacterial flora. Therefore, after taking antibiotics it is important to restore and maintain the good bacterial flora with probiotics. The most common good bacteria is L. acidophilus but there are many others. The best probiotic products will contain from seven to fifteen different strains of bacteria. They also contain prebiotics that nourish the good bacteria. Unfortunately, much of the probiotics may be killed by harsh stomach acids while passing through the stomach. Some probiotic brands treat the probiotics to prevent this kill-off and perhaps also provide timed release. Probiotics are also found in yogurt so eating a serving of, preferably plain, yogurt is another means of maintaining the good bacterial flora. Probiotics have been found to promote regularity and reduce flatulence.

After the stomach empties the food and juice mixture into the small intestine, the juices of the two other digestive organs mix with the food. One of these organs, the pancreas, produces a juice that contains a wide array of enzymes to break down the carbohydrates, fats, and proteins in food. Other enzymes that are active in the process come from glands in the wall of the intestine.

The second organ, the liver, produces yet another digestive juice— bile. Bile is stored between meals in the gallbladder. At mealtime, it is squeezed out of the gallbladder, through the bile ducts, and into the intestine to mix with the fat in food. The bile acids dissolve fat into the watery contents of the intestine, much like detergents that dissolve grease from a frying pan. After fat is dissolved, it is digested by enzymes from the pancreas and the lining of the intestine.

Absorption and Transport of Nutrients

Most digested molecules of food, as well as water and minerals, are absorbed through the small intestine. The mucosa of the small intestine contains many folds that are covered with tiny fingerlike projections called villi. In turn, the villi are covered with microscopic projections called microvilli. These structures create a vast surface area through which nutrients can be absorbed. Specialized cells allow absorbed materials to cross the mucosa into the blood, where they are carried off in the bloodstream to other parts of the body for storage or further chemical change. This part of the process varies with different types of nutrients.

Carbohydrates, The *Dietary Guidelines for Americans 2005* recommend that 45 to 65 percent of total daily calories be from carbohydrates. Foods rich in carbohydrates include bread, potatoes, dried peas and beans, rice, pasta, fruits, and vegetables. Many of these foods contain both starch and fiber.

The digestible carbohydrates—starch and sugar—are broken into simpler molecules by enzymes in the saliva, in juice produced by the pancreas, and in the lining of the small intestine. Starch is digested in two steps. First, an enzyme in the saliva and pancreatic juice breaks the starch into molecules called maltose. Then an enzyme in the lining of the small intestine splits the maltose into glucose molecules that can be absorbed into the blood. Glucose is carried through the bloodstream to the liver, where it is stored or used to provide energy for the work of the body.

Sugars are digested in one step. An enzyme in the lining of the small intestine digests sucrose, also known as table sugar, into glucose and fructose, which are absorbed through the intestine into the blood. Milk contains another type of sugar, lactose, which is changed into absorbable molecules by another enzyme in the intestinal lining.

Fiber is indigestible and moves through the digestive tract without being broken down by enzymes. Many foods contain both soluble and insoluble fiber. Soluble fiber dissolves easily in water and takes on a soft, gel-like texture in the intestines. Insoluble fiber, on the other hand, passes essentially unchanged through the intestines.

Fiber gives us a feeling of fullness when we are eating. It also cleanses the intestines and colon as it passes through them. The gummy substance produced by insoluble fiber binds cholesterol and carbohydrates and inhibits blood sugar levels. Sources of insoluble fiber are bran, cereals, brown rice, and popcorn; fruits such as apples and berries; and vegetables such as potatoes (both white and sweet), peas, beets, carrots, and asparagus.

Soluble fiber soaks up water and facilitates the passage of food through the intestines. Good sources of soluble fiber are fruits such as apricots, plums, apples, strawberries and mangos; also barley, psyllium and legumes (dry beans and peas). Good vegetable sources are the cabbage family, broccoli, and brussel sprouts, as well as carrots, turnips, and white potatoes. Some foods contain both soluble and insoluble fiber.

Protein. Foods such as meat, eggs, and beans consist of giant molecules of protein that must be digested by enzymes before they can be used to build and repair body tissues. An enzyme in the juice of the stomach starts the digestion of swallowed protein. Then in the small intestine, several enzymes from the pancreatic juice and the lining of the intestine complete the breakdown of huge protein molecules into small molecules called amino acids. These small molecules can be absorbed through the small intestine into the blood and then be carried to all parts of the body to build the walls and other parts of cells.

Fats. Fat molecules are a rich source of energy for the body. The first step in digestion of a fat such as butter is to dissolve it into the watery content of the intestine. The bile acids produced by the liver dissolve fat into tiny droplets and allow pancreatic and intestinal enzymes to break the large fat molecules into smaller ones. Some of these small molecules are fatty acids and cholesterol. The bile acids combine with the fatty acids and cholesterol and help these molecules move into the cells of the mucosa. Inside these cells, the small molecules are formed back into large ones, most of which pass into vessels called lymphatics near the intestine. These small vessels carry the reformed fat to the veins of the chest, and the blood carries the fat to storage depots in different parts of the body.

Many people have supposed that they could lose fat or avoid adding fat to their bodies by simply eliminating fat from their diets. One reason this is difficult to do is that it's fat that gives food its good flavor. Another reason is that it's virtually impossible to eliminate all fat because fats occur naturally in various forms in the food we eat.

Finally, it's undesirable to eliminate all fat from our diet because fat is our principle source of energy. Felicia Busch, in her book *Nutrition Secrets*, explains:

"Fats are really combinations of many different fatty acids, and each one differently affects how your body works. With nine calories per gram, fat is the most concentrated energy source in food. Fat is critical for growth in children, is required for healthy skin, helps hormone-like substances regulate body processes, and is essential for the absorption of fat-soluble vitamins."[12] There are four basic types of fats that we must concern ourselves with.

Monounsaturated fat is the healthiest form of fat to have in the diet. This includes olive oil, which actually is a combination of monounsaturated, polyunsaturated and saturated fatty acids. They are the healthiest because they break down most easily yielding their nutrients to our bodies without causing arterial plaque.

Saturated fat is one that we need to watch out for because it can increase our blood cholesterol levels. However, we need some fat, so rather than totally eliminating it we should keep it to a minimum. If total fat is five percent and saturated fat is three percent that is acceptable. Saturated fat also raises our good (HDL) Cholesterol levels. So, if a label indicates that it does not exceed ten percent, that is reasonable. If it is above that be cautious to use it very sparingly in your diet. Animal products such as meat and dairy are the basic sources of high saturated fat, but it is also found in some tree oils.

Trans fats are manufactured by changing an unsaturated oil by adding hydrogen to it. This is the most harmful of the fat sources; it can seriously increase the bad (LDL) cholesterol blood levels which causes plaque in our arteries leading to heart diseases. Because it enhances the flavor of a product, manufacturers have added it to many products. If a product's ingredient list includes hydrogenated oil or partly hydrogenated oil, you should avoid that product. Fortunately, due to its bad reputation, many producers are now eliminating it from their products and restaurants are ceasing from using these oils.

Polyunsaturated fats, as the name (poly) suggests, have many bonds and are liquid at room temperature. These have not been found to be particularly harmful in the diet. Because they have a high smoke point, they are useful for cooking which requires high temperatures. These uses are not included in the longevity diet.

Vitamins. Other vital components of food that are absorbed through the small intestine are vitamins. The two types of vitamins are classified by the fluid in which they can be dissolved: water-soluble vitamins (all the B vitamins and vitamin C) and fat-soluble vitamins (vitamins A, D, E, and K). Fat-soluble vitamins are stored in the liver and fatty tissue of the body, but water-soluble vitamins are not easily stored and excess amounts of them are flushed out in the urine.

Water and salt. Most of the material absorbed through the small intestine is water in which salt is dissolved. The salt and water come from the food and liquid you swallow and the juices secreted by the many digestive glands.

How is the digestive process controlled?

Regulators

The major hormones that control the functions of the digestive system are produced and released by cells in the mucosa of the stomach and small intestine.

These hormones are released into the blood of the digestive tract, travel back to the heart and through the arteries, and return to the digestive system where they stimulate digestive juices and cause organ movement. The main hormones that control digestion are gastrin, secretin, and cholecystokinin (CCK):

Gastrin causes the stomach to produce an acid for dissolving and digesting some foods. Gastrin is also necessary for normal cell growth in the lining of the stomach, small intestine, and colon.

Secretin causes the pancreas to send out a digestive juice that is rich in bicarbonate. The bicarbonate helps neutralize the acidic stomach contents as they enter the small intestine. Secretin also stimulates the stomach to produce pepsin, an enzyme that digests protein, and stimulates the liver to produce bile.

CCK causes the pancreas to produce the enzymes of pancreatic juice, and causes the gallbladder to empty. It also promotes normal cell growth of the pancreas.

Additional hormones in the digestive system regulate appetite:

Ghrelin is produced in the stomach and upper intestine in the absence of food in the digestive system and stimulates appetite.

Peptide. Both of these hormones work on the brain to help regulate the intake of food for energy. According to researchers at Albert Einstein College of Medicine of Yeshiva University, specialized nerve cells in the hypothalamus of the brain sense whether the body contains adequate amounts of nutrients and stored body fat. The cells send out messages through nutrient sensitive pathways telling other parts of the brain to adjust food intake, metabolic rates and physical activity to balance caloric intake with calories burned.

Nerve Regulators

Two types of nerves help control the action of the digestive system.

Extrinsic, or outside, nerves come to the digestive organs from the brain or the spinal cord. They release two chemicals, acetylcholine and adrenaline. Acetylcholine causes the muscle layer of the digestive organs to squeeze with more force, increasing the speed of food and juice passing through the digestive tract. It also causes the stomach and pancreas to produce more digestive juice. Adrenaline has the opposite effect; it relaxes the muscle of the stomach and intestine and decreases the flow of blood to these organs, slowing or stopping digestion.

The intrinsic, or inside, nerves make up a very dense network embedded in the walls of the esophagus, stomach, small intestine, and colon. The intrinsic nerves are triggered to act when the walls of the hollow organs are stretched by food. They release many different substances that speed up or delay the movement of food and the production of juices by the digestive organs.

Together, nerves, hormones, the blood, and the organs of the digestive system conduct the complex tasks of digesting and absorbing nutrients from the foods and liquids you consume each day.

Chapter Five
Weight Loss With The Longevity Diet

Anyone who seriously follows The Longevity Diet will naturally lose weight. To do that you must make a firm commitment and set a goal to succeed. All that has been presented up to this point has been to help you understand the essentials of weight loss and healthy living for longevity. Maintaining a strong immune system with regard to appropriate hormone levels is essential for success. All of the steps of the plan that are presented here must be adequately observed to get the most from The Longevity Diet and fully succeed in living long and living well. Keep in mind that the plan is for a lifestyle leading to your goal and the prize you desire.

You will achieve many benefits from setting your will to shed your extra pounds. If you have an aching back, it may be from being unbalanced from carrying too much fat on your belly. Shedding that excess fat will not only relieve your back but potentially add years to your life by reducing bodily stress and your risk of disease. Relieving that stress will lead to greater health.

Packing extra weight around your mid-section is also a risk factor for bladder control problems which may be alleviated by losing weight. Another benefit of achieving optimal body mass is that it lifts your spirit and makes you feel better about yourself and life. . The world will just look a lot different to you with your new body. You will feel better and be more interested and capable of doing things that are satisfying to you. Optimal body mass is calculated by dividing a person's weight in kilograms by his or her height in squared meters. It is preferable to have an index figure under 30.

From our studies of centenarian people, we have noticed some things about their eating habits that we believe contribute to their healthy body mass and hence to their longevity. The first thing that we notice is that people who live long eat small portions and avoid overeating. To achieve this, they may eat from small dishes. A modest portion on a large plate may not look like much, but on a small plate it appears to be a satisfying amount. There is a psychological factor working here.

The next thing is that they learn to commit themselves to pushing back from the table when they feel about ¾ full. They have learned that when they feel totally full they have actually overeaten. It takes a while for the sensation of fullness to register in the brain. When beginning this practice the urge to eat more may be there and one must learn to resist. It is a physical fact that, when an individual practices eating less, the stomach, in time, adjusts to the smaller portions. If there is an urge for more, drinking some water helps to fill the void without adding calories.

People who are very active, work hard physically and burn a lot of energy during the day may require larger meals. The point here is to adjust your eating habits to your true energy needs rather than your desires. Eating "see food" (whatever looks good) is not healthy eating.

When eating it is best to take small bites, eat slowly, chew your food thoroughly, and savor your meal. This aids the digestive process. Eating with good company and enjoyable conversation helps to achieve this goal. While it's not generally advisable to eat in front of the TV, it may be the best substitute for one living alone.

If you feel an urge to snack between meals, try drinking some water instead. The urge you feel may actually be for water instead of food. If convenient, you may also drink a cup of green tea sweetened with an appropriate sweetener. However, if you need an energy boost between meals, try eating a granola bar, an apple, or another fruit.

Many people have developed a habit of eating a snack late in the evening. This is strictly a habit that individuals should strive to overcome. Some accommodate the desire for eating with the learned habit of eating while watching TV. This is an unhealthy association. Perhaps reading in the evening may help to break the habit. There are products on the market that will help control the urge to eat. Before resorting to one of these, an individual must be aware that an idle or stressed mind may turn to food for satisfaction. If this is the cause of the seeming hunger, you should address the true need. If you have the desire to eat in the late evening, try taking a drink of water and going to bed earlier. The extra rest will be beneficial to you. It is said that every hour of rest before midnight is worth two hours after midnight. You and your spouse may find that you appreciate the extra time spent in closeness.

If you feel the need to use a supplement to accelerate your weight loss goals we suggest a new product that Life Extension has recently made available. This product is called *Calorie Control Weight Management Formula.* This formula is a berry-pomegranate flavored powder that is mixed with water 15-30 minutes before the two largest meals of the day. It contains four ingredients that have been proven to be helpful. The first is a fiber called LuraLean that swells in the stomach to help reduce calorie consumption. The second is an extract, *Phaseolus vulgaris,* of the white kidney bean that aids breaking down carbohydrates in the digestive tract. Third, is a plant extract referred to as Irvinga that helps to decrease appetite. Fourth is a green tea phytosome that absorbs well in the bloodstream to boost your metabolic resting rate. In a clinical study, users of this last ingredient have been found to lose as much as 30.1 pounds of weight in a 90 day period.

It is suggested that you seriously try The Longevity Diet alone before resorting to the expense of this, or any, supplement because following the diet with balanced meals will provide the same functions, although it may take a while longer. The downsides of the supplement are the expense and the inconvenience of needing to remember to take it faithfully before meals. Less expensive aids for weight loss are Tonalin CLA (conjugated linoleic acid) and, particularly useful for diabetic persons, are chromium picolinate and cinnamon. Using The Longevity Diet, this author has exceeded his weight loss goal by losing 70 pounds and five inches from his waist, thus achieving a very acceptable body mass ratio. I have lots of vim, vigor and vitality and appear younger than my age.

> "The truth is, the only way to eat what we want and lose
> weight is to want what causes weight loss. In other words,
> our desires have to change before diets will work. The
> desire to be thin is not enough; we must also desire what
> is good for us – nutritious foods and plenty of exercise."[13]
>
> Julie Ackerman Link

Chapter Six
Nutrition, Vitamins and Supplements for the Longevity Diet

Some doctors and others believe that it is not necessary to take vitamins, minerals, and herbal supplements. They maintain that a person <u>can</u> get enough of these nutrients from their daily diet. Note the underlined word <u>can</u>. Ideally, that would be possible, but we don't live in an ideal world. The land where most of our food is raised has been continuously cropped for many years. This procedure has depleted the soil of some of its naturally available nutrient, and if they are not in the soil they will not be sufficiently available in the harvested produce that you buy at the market.

Most of these croplands are fertilized with chemical fertilizers. Home gardeners that organically fertilize their gardens attest to the superiority of the vegetables they raise. For this reason, The Longevity Diet advises home gardening whenever possible. But be sure to fertilize your garden with organic mulch and manure. If space is limited, consider using the border around the foundation of the home or use planters on the patio. Seek whatever space you can find. An alternative is to buy produce from an organic gardener. Another consideration is that due to seasonal availability, some fresh vegetables and fruits may not always be available to be included in the diet. Taking vitamins daily helps to fill the void.

Those who are taking vitamins, minerals, and herbal supplements are increasing in number each year. This number includes many doctors who are realizing the need. Perhaps you could ask your doctor what he or she takes. The answer may surprise you. How do you think doctors stay healthy when they are seeing sick people all the time? A doctor who has a heart problem will begin taking supplements to support the heart but may rarely suggest an alternative such as supplements to a patient. People who take supplements find that they have stronger immune systems to help them stay healthy as well as more energy to enjoy life.

On the supplement container, you will see an RDA (Recommended Daily Allowance) figure. Ongoing research has revealed that this figure is minimal at best, and often too low. However, those who set the RDA are slow to make adjustments in their recommendations. Therefore, we must take the advice of researchers and doctors that keep up-to-date on our real need for various nutrients. What is suggested here is believed to be adequate for the average adult. There may be times when an extra-large dose of a nutrient is called for. For example, some doctors may inject a giant mega-dose of vitamin C to aid a person in quickly overcoming a serious respiratory problem. As a one-time occurrence, this is entirely safe. It is possible to get too much of a good thing, but this does not usually happen with the doses that most people take, even when they increase the dosage for a short time, as some do with vitamin C or D to manage a health crisis.

Every adult should daily take a multiple vitamin-mineral supplement. Look for an *Ultra Vitamin and Mineral Combination* or *Whole Food Vitamin and Mineral Supplement*. Typically these contain vitamins, essential minerals, and trace elements, and some have herbal ingredients included. The formula should have 10,000 IU of vitamin A, preferably in the form of beta-carotene, as well as all of the B vitamins, vitamins C, D, etc. The vitamin A content is the first indication of the quality of the vitamin product. The best formulations are not usually available at a pharmacy or department store. A health food store may have a good product, but it will likely be expensive. You may find it more economical to purchase your vitamin and other supplement needs from manufacturers or dealers that are available online or by phone. You will find some of these in the reference section in the back of this book.

The multiple vitamin – mineral may not have an adequate amount of some nutrients, with the exception of vitamin A, so, in addition to the multiple vitamin and mineral, you may want to add an extra dose of some supplements to assure an adequate intake of certain nutrients. Listed here are some of the most essential supplements for longevity with a description of their functions. All are important, but some will be provided in adequate amounts in the multiple vitamin – mineral combination. Individual circumstances may control requirements.

We have noted that the Japanese people who are known for their longevity include in their diet quantities of **seaweed.** Being a nation of many islands, fresh seaweed is available to them. Fortunately, it is also widely available as a food supplement. Seaweed contains an abundant amount of vitamins and minerals and therefore seaweed, including brown seaweed, kelp, dulse seaweed, and red algea in combination with spirulina (blue-green algea) and chlorella (especially split cell chlorella), may be a suitable alternative for a multiple vitamin. It is not wise or cost effective to double-up on vitamins and seaweed contains large amounts of vitamins A, C, and B12. Additionally seaweed contains varying amounts of sodium, calcium, magnesium, potassium, chlorine, sulfur, phosphorus, iron, zinc, copper, selenium, fluoride, manganese, boron, nickel, and cobalt. One of the best things about seaweed is that it is a primary source of iodine, which is necessary to the thyroid, breasts, and prostate and is known to prevent the growth of cancer cells. A healthy thyroid has been found to be essential to the health of the body in many respects. Seaweed also contains folate which is vital for the creation of new body cells. It can easily penetrate the membranes of all body cells. Notably, being fat soluble, folate has great ability to cross the blood brain barrier and protect the cells of the brain to inhibit cognitive decline and improve memory and concentration.

The nutrients in seaweed provide anti-oxidant protection, are anti-inflammatory, have a blood thinning effect that aides circulation, reduce LDL cholesterol (thus improving cardiovascular health), helps to maintain healthy blood sugar levels, and supports weight loss. All of this makes seaweed a super food that the Japanese have wisely learned to avail themselves of.

Vitamin A – Take at least 10,000 IU daily, preferably as beta-carotene. This vitamin helps to maintain a strong immune system that will fight cold and flu viruses, and it can help to clear sinus problems. It promotes healthy skin and is good for our vision, including our night vision. In fact, it supports all of our senses. It is a protection against heart disease, high blood pressure, and stroke, and the beta-carotene makes it a potent cancer fighter, especially for lung, colon, prostate, and uterine cancers but also for every other kind. Vitamin A has also been found to counteract the adverse effects of all kinds of stress including that caused by environmental pollutants. We cannot overestimate the value of this vitamin for those at any stage of life, but it is especially vital for aging people who are more susceptible to disease states. Some of the best sources with beta-carotene content are carrots, sweet potatoes, dark green leafy vegetables, winter squash, cantaloupes, and apricots. Broccoli is also an excellent source of this vitamin.

Vitamin B Complex as B50 or B100: If you take B50 you will want to take one two times each day. If you take B100, only one each day may be sufficient unless you have a special need for these.

The B Complex vitamins include:

B1, Thiamin: This vitamin supports the brain and nervous system functions including aiding memory, repressing depression, and enhancing initiative and concentration.

B$_2$, Riboflavin: This is known to lengthen the life of red blood cells and assist folate in producing new red blood cells in bone marrow. It may also help prevent cataract formation. Yogurt is a good source.

Niacin: This vitamin relieves arthritis symptoms and depression while it aids sleep and relaxation.

B6: As little as 10 mg of this vitamin taken with at least 200 mg of magnesium prevents kidney stone formation. It also inhibits blood clotting, supports the heart by helping to prevent LDL cholesterol buildup, and relieves the symptoms of PMS (Premenstral Stress Syndrome). It's needed by women using oral birth control products. Those with adequate levels have less irritability, restlessness, and fatigue. Good food sources are wheat products such as bread, crackers, cereal, and whole wheat pasta.

B12: This vitamin supports the nervous system and is instrumental in red blood cell production. It can be inhibited by many prescription drugs prescribed for blood pressure, Parkinson's disease, and cholesterol.

Folate (folic acid): This is essential for red blood cell formation; it also prevents anemia, fatigue, and restless legs and helps prevent depression.

Women of child bearing age need to take this, especially if they are using oral birth control. A good natural source is leafy green vegetables. It's abundant in spinach but is destroyed by cooking.

Pantothenate: This vitamin is needed throughout the body to build coenzyme A (CoA), which is a necessary catalyst that helps convert fats, carbohydrates, and proteins into energy. It has been found to be useful in relieving the symptoms of some allergies, especially hay fever, and prevents fatigue. Dr. Roger Williams, Ph.D. has found experimentally that an adequate amount of this vitamin may add as much as 10 years to a person's life.

Para-aminobenzoic acid (PABA): It protects the skin from ultraviolet rays of the sun. This vitamin should not be taken with antibiotics as it can cancel their effectiveness.

Choline (KO-leen): Primarily aids the memory and may help to eliminate "senior moments".

Inositol: Helps prevent nerve damage.

Biotin: Aids digestion by helping to release energy from foods and helps create healthy skin and nails.

Vitamin C: We think of this vitamin mostly with regard to its ability to relieve or ward off the effects of colds and flu, however, it has many more uses in our bodies. In addition to giving a major boost to the immune system, it is a powerful antioxidant. When there is sickness or injury to the body, it speeds the healing process. It also provides strong protection against cardiovascular disease, reducing the possibility of a heart attack or reducing the damage from such an event. In patients who have high cholesterol, it may reduce it. Taken in mega doses, it acts as an antibiotic to the respiratory system and can greatly accelerate recuperation from sickness.

Other benefits of taking a daily dose of this vitamin include assisting the healing process of cancer patients, protecting the kidneys from damage and ameliorating asthma. Vitamin C has even been found helpful in increasing bone density.

Vitamin C is abundant in citrus fruit, but it also occurs naturally in guava, strawberries, black currants, many other fruits, and even some vegetables. Taken as a daily supplement, 1000-2000 mg (divided into two daily doses) is recommended. The form of Ester-C may be easier to use than other forms because this form provides a buffer against stomach upset due to the acidity.

Vitamin D: This has been referred to as the sunshine vitamin, but it is difficult for people in the latitudes north of Tuscon, Arizona to get an adequate amount from that source. Even in latitudes from Tuscon southward if people are fully clothed and wear hats they may not get enough vitamin D. Many people in these sunny latitudes tend to seek protection from the sun as much as possible. It has been found that the skin of older adults cannot produce sufficient amounts of D3 even with adequate exposure which makes supplementation even more important for these individuals.

Many studies resulting in new discoveries have been completed in recent years revealing the great importance of this vitamin and of the effective amount needed daily by individuals. Vitamin D_3 is essential to healthy functioning of the immune system and is also considered to be helpful in controlling inflammation. For the prevention of flu, it can be more effective than a flu shot. Studies show that it may be helpful in the prevention and treatment of prostate, colon, breast, skin, and possibly other cancers. Adequate amounts may also be helpful in preventing diabetes. Still other studies have indicated possible helpfulness of D_3 in treating depression and mental disorders. Many who are afflicted with Parkinson's disease have an insufficient level of this vitamin. There are different forms of vitamin D, but D3 is the best one to use because it remains in the blood for up to 30 days and has proven to be the most potent form.

Some competent doctors, including Dr. Jonathan V. Wright of the Tahoma Clinic, now recommend that the adult dose should be 4000 to 8000 IU daily. The average dosage is 5,000 IU. When the body is stressed by sickness such as the flu, it is safe to take up to 50,000 IU per day for a short time (one–three days). Mega dosing for very long can cause toxicity, which may be detected by symptoms such as nausea. In larger dosages, this vitamin seems to act like an antibiotic. Older people who are deficient in this vitamin may be susceptible to disease states. Researchers at Johns Hopkins discovered that vitamin D deficiency was related to a 26% increase in death from any cause in the study group over the nine years of the study. The research points out the magnitude of this vitamin's value to an individual's health and longevity.

Vitamin D$_3$ helps to improve bone density by facilitating the absorption of calcium into the bones, and it works best when taken in conjunction with adequate amounts of calcium. It also protects the heart from disease, working best with coenzyme Q10 and other vitamins and minerals. A deficiency of D3 is recognized as a main cause of osteoporosis in women. This vitamin works best in conjunction with adequate amounts of calcium. It has also been found to be of great importance to protect the heart from disease. In this instance it works best with coenzyme Q10 and other vitamins and minerals. Considering the widespread deficiency and all of the new findings that are continually being revealed by research into the need for this vitamin it is strongly advisable to supplement with D3 to assure adequate protection.

Vitamin E: This essential vitamin has an oil base that coats the platelets of blood preventing them from clotting together. As such it is, for many, a much safer alternative to Coumadin. Angina sufferers appreciate its benefits. It is also a very effective antioxidant. It works in conjunction with vitamin A to prevent oxidation, so it can lessen the negative effects of air pollution and other stress factors. It may even help to eliminate mercury from the body. Many hand and body lotions contain vitamin E because of its well-known benefit to the skin.

Other benefits of vitamin E are that it helps to balance the (bad) LDL cholesterol with the (good) HDL cholesterol. It helps to overcome the tendency to get leg cramps, and it is very effective in wound healing. Those facing surgery need this vitamin. Some break the capsule open and squeeze the oil onto the wound to retard the itching of the healing process. Some claim it has helped relieve shingles and arthritis. If that is not reason enough to take E supplements we will add that it may also help to prevent cataracts, improve immunity against infections, and it works synergistically with anticancer drugs enhancing the effectiveness of the drug.

The best natural sources of E include almonds, hazelnuts, peanut butter, wheat germ, and rice bran. It is very difficult to eat enough to get sufficient E through diet alone, so supplementing is very important. The usual effective dose is 400-800 IUs. It's important to use the most effective form, gamma E with mixed tocopherols or natural d-alpha tocopherol acetate. Absorption of vitamin E is diminished by antacids, so if you take these you will need a heftier dose of E.

Dr. Denham Harman, M.D., of the University of Nebraska College of Medicine agrees with many other doctors and scientists that free radicals are a main cause of aging and that by taking antioxidants like vitamin E a person may add many years to her or his life. He said that including vitamin E in the diet "may reasonably be expected to add five to ten or more years of healthy, productive life to the life span of the average person"[14]

Vitamin K is best known for its role in controlling the clotting factor of our blood. Without ample vitamin K, a person could bleed to death from an injury. Vitamin K "thickens" the blood, so individuals using Coumadin, a blood thinner, should be cautious of how much K they have. Individuals need to have a balance between "thick" and "thin" blood.

There are two forms of vitamin K. The first is K1, which is derived from green leafy vegetables, and the second is K2 which is found primarily in dairy products. Of these two forms, K2 is the most desired, the most bioactive, and the hardest to get an ample supply of from our food. Some K1 is changed to K2 in the intestines, but, it is best to take a supplement to assure an ample supply in the bloodstream. Vitamin K2 is absorbed well from supplements when taken with meals containing some fat. This is one reason why we need some fat in our diets.

Vitamin K has some other benefits that are especially important to aging adults. We have long known that vitamin D is important for the proper functioning of calcium in our bodies, but now we know that it also takes vitamin K for proper calcium metabolism. Calcium is important to prevent bone thinning, promote strong bones, and prevent osteoporosis. However, calcium is also responsible for calcification (atherosclerosis) in our arteries. Without an adequate amount of vitamin K, an inappropriate amount of calcium accumulates in our arteries, leaving a deficiency in our bones. Thus, vitamin K2 is like a traffic cop protecting the arteries and heart by directing the calcium to the bones.

There has been no indication of side effects in the use of vitamin K so it is believed to be safe. Dosages may vary from 50 mcg to 1000 mcg. Considering that it is safe and has very important benefits for older men and women, a high dosage in the form of K2 is recommended.

Resveratrol is the key supplement in an anti-aging program aimed at helping individuals to live long, disease-free, enjoyable lives. It is a great benefit to individuals in boosting gene expression as it enhances genetic pathways, leading to higher quality of life and longer life span. Caloric restriction is one of the best ways to control obesity and promote longevity. Resveratrol seems to mimic caloric restriction. Resveratrol significantly reduces the risk of death from a high calorie diet. Therefore, those who can control calorie intake by using The Longevity Diet but who also take resveratrol have a tremendous boost toward achieving their longevity goals.

Resveratrol is believed to be effective in combating numerous diseases including heart problems, cancer, diabetes, Alzheimer's and neurological problems. This is attributed to its powerful antioxidant and anti-inflammatory effects which controls free radicals and inflammation. It is likely that further studies will reveal more fully the benefits to be derived from this supplement. It is most highly recommended to be included in every adult diet, especially that of those from mid-life upward of those who may be disease prone.

Resveratrol first gained attention as scientists studied the "French Paradox". It was noticed that people in Southern France had a lower incidence of heart disease than other cultures although they ate a rich high fat diet which should subject them to this disease. It was believed that their consumption of red wine was the reason for this paradox. Red wine is made from grapes that have a high resveratrol content. Due to changing horticultural methods, the content is not as high as it had been in earlier times. Other plants, including Japanese knotweed, berries, and even peanuts, are also sources of resveratrol. Supplements are the best way to get your resveratrol because a person would have to drink at least 41 glasses of red wine to equal the daily dosage of resveratrol. Daily dosages of resveratrol may be as great as 250 mg. The larger dosages have been found to be safe, but even lower dosages seem to be effective.

"Dr. Richard A. Miller of the University of Michigan speculates that with effects similar to caloric restriction, resveratrol could extend human longevity to about 112 or even 140 years of healthy life"[15] .

Acetyl-L-carnitine arginate is the best of about eight various forms of carnitine. It improves mood, memory, and cognition. It enhances energy production in the brain and in cells throughout the body. Although it protects all body cells against age-related degeneration, its most important functions are in the brain. There it works in conjunction with CoQ10 (100-300 mg) and alpha lipoic acid (250-500 mg) to maintain mitochondrial functioning. Degenerative diseases are a certain consequence of diminishing mitochondrial functioning. It also promotes the growth of neurites in the brain. By facilitating the synthesis of acetylcholine, an important neurotransmitter, it nourishes and provides cognitive support to the nervous system. Further, it enhances the release of dopamine and aids in binding it to dopamine receptors. As such it may be helpful in preventing dementia, Alzheimers and may also help those with Parkinson's disease.

This is a very important nutrient for aging adults. The daily dose for prevention is 1,000 – 2,000 mg per day. Those with neurological problems should take 3,000 mg daily or another amount as directed by a doctor.

Alpha lipoic acid in its most biologically active form is R-lipoic acid. This is the form that the body produces to enhance its body functions, and it is the most potent antioxidant supporting mitochondrial functions. It also is supportive of inflammatory responses. It boosts the activity of some other supplements such as carnitine and DHEA. The dosage is up to 600 mg daily.

Ginkgo biloba is one of the most ancient herbal extracts; it has been used by the Chinese for over twenty centuries. The tree from which the leaves come is itself one of the oldest known living things. There must be something about its longevity that can aid our longevity. The extract contains several antioxidants, making it very effective at controlling free radical activity. It is also believed to aid circulation, particularly circulation to the brain, and support brain function by carrying oxygen to the brain, aiding memory. It is another supporter of the mitochondria of our body cells. It is also thought that it may help relieve the effects of tinnitus.

One of its functions is as a blood thinner which has two consequences; it can promote excess bleeding when an individual is injured, and it should not be used in conjunction with other blood thinners. It is important for healthy individuals to take not more than 120 mg per day. The upside of this is that it is helpful to prevent blood clotting.

L-arginine is an essential amino acid needed for the production of nitric oxide. It tends to dilate blood vessels, so it is sometimes used in preparations for erectile dysfunction. It aids wound healing by increasing protein synthesis, which also increases cellular replication. It helps to remove excess ammonia from the body and may assist the function of the immune system.

Arginine has an effect upon the release of growth hormone. In this function it works with ornithine. There is some concern that increases in growth hormone stimulated by arginine could negatively affect the pancreas. Supplementation is usually only needed in times of stress as the body tends to make its own supply. Dairy products, fish, nuts, and chocolate are good food sources. There is reason to be cautious about taking supplemental arginine because in high doses it has been found to stimulate cancer growth. But again, for people with cancer it can combat it by stimulating the immune system.

CoenzymeQ10 (CoQ10) is a compound that occurs naturally in the body and is essential for producing cellular energy. It is especially crucial to the health of the cardiovascular and immune systems.

CoQ10 is foremost known for its ability to prevent or control many various heart problems. High blood pressure is an indicator of the possibility of these problems. The inability of blood vessels to transport sufficient blood flow is the root of the problems. CoQ10 has been found to aid the circulation of blood through the vessels. CoQ10 is incompatible with some statin drugs which tend to deplete blood levels of the nutrient.

There are many other applications where CoQ10 has been found helpful. It supports the immune system in several circumstances. It may modify the effects of allergic conditions, including asthma and hay fever. There are indications that it may help those with HIV infections; it has been found to reduce the frequency of migraine headaches, and it may slow the progression of Parkinson's disease. Additionally, it is another nutrient that is an antioxidant.

We cannot overlook that CoQ10 can potentially play an important role in the prevention of prostate and breast cancers as well as aiding recuperation after chemotherapy. It has been found to hinder cancerous cells while having no negative effect on healthy cells. It seems to have great potential for preventing lethal melanoma skin cancers and is included in many skin creams.

CoQ10 is often needed by aging individuals because the natural production within the body declines as people grow older. The rate of decline can vary with individuals, but it may begin even before mid-life. For supplementation CoQ10 can be found in two forms. The first is ubiquinone, which is an artificial form. More recently, scientists have learned to duplicate the bioidentical natural form, which is ubiquinol. The latter is the preferred form to use. The most effective form of ubiquinol is believed to be Kaneka QH. It is available in dosages of 50-200 mg. Unless a medical practitioner directs differently follow the directions on the label.

Magnesium is one of the most prominent and biochemically active minerals in the body. It has hundreds of functions to perform which make it totally essential to maintain at an adequate level. Studies have shown that those with the highest intake of magnesium have the lowest incidence of type 2 diabetes. It may also provide protection against metabolic syndrome. There are many ways in which it is implicated as essential for cardiovascular health. It can help regulate blood pressure, prevent arrhythmia, reduce the risk of angina and is particularly helpful in saving the lives of individuals with congestive heart failure.

"The risks for ischemic stroke are pretty much the same as risk factors for heart attacks. Essentially, low magnesium levels increase the risk of ischemic stroke. A 10 year study of 2,183 men in Wales found those eating diets low in magnesium had a fifty percent higher risk of sudden death from heart attacks than those eating one third more magnesium".[16]

It has been discovered that a deficiency of magnesium may be responsible for the increased incidence of forgetfulness (senior moments or worse) as men and women become older. In other words deficiency keeps the synapses from connecting. Considering how disconcerting this is for seniors it is an important reason to maintain an optimal level of this mineral to reduce these occurrences. Also, with regard to mental functions magnesium prevents or eases the incidence of migraine headaches.

A new form of magnesium, Magnesium-L-Threonate, has recently been developed that is especially effective in aiding brain functions including both long-term and short-term memory. This is possible because magnesium-L-threonate has the ability to cross the blood-brain barrier. Studies have indicated that it may also aid learning and improve mood. Because this development is so new, studies are ongoing to verify the usefulness of this form of magnesium.

Because about sixty percent per cent of the magnesium in the body is in the bones, it is obvious that it is essential for healthy, strong bones. This indicates it as being important in preventing osteoporosis and bone thinning. Deficits have been associated with asthma, anxiety, and colon cancer. It may take some time for the effects of deficiencies to become evident. Medications such as antibiotics and diuretics can create a deficiency, so extra supplementation may be needed when taking these.

Magnesium is available in various forms; most notably magnesium oxide, magnesium citrate, and magnesium aspartate. For restoring a chemical imbalance, the aspartate or citrate forms are preferable. There are formulations available that contain all three forms. Magnesium is a natural calcium blocker. Therefore, calcium intake should be balanced with magnesium. Cal-Mag formulas are available that have the correct balance. In 1974 Harvard researchers discovered that 300 mg per day of magnesium with 10 mg of vitamin B6 is a preventive for calcium oxalate kidney stones.

The importance of magnesium cannot be overemphasized. While it is generally safe, excessively large doses, which rarely occur, can cause nausea, abdominal cramping, diarrhea, weakness, and loss of appetite. The current recommended dose is 500 mg daily for men and 400 mg for women. Natural sources of magnesium are nuts, whole grains, legumes, dark green leafy vegetables, salmon, and trout.

Zinc is an indispensible mineral for healthy body functioning. The natural sources include nuts, oatmeal, and bran. However, most soil in the United States is deficient in zinc and so also are foods raised in it. Therefore, supplementation is essential for persons to get an adequate amount in their diets.

Zinc has many applications in the body. One of the most important is its usefulness in proper immune function. When the cold and flu season comes, zinc helps to protect us from these viruses. Zinc lozenges are very useful to soothe throat irritations and help to shorten the duration of these ailments. In aging adults, it helps maintain functioning of the thymus gland, which is the most important gland in the immune system, although this gland may not be functioning at one hundred percent capacity.

Zinc also functions as an antioxidant, helps to control inflammation, and is helpful to prevent certain types of cancers. It is important for normal human growth and development with regard to height, weight, and the production of healthy sperm.

For men, zinc is essential to maintain a healthy prostate. Unfortunately, most men don't think about this until they have urinary problems. The ureter passes through the prostate, so consequently when the prostate becomes enlarged from BPH (benign prostate hypertrophy) it becomes difficult, and sometimes impossible, to urinate. A symptom of the problem is frequent trips to the bathroom and a weak, meager urine flow, making it difficult to fully empty the bladder. If this is caused, even partly, by a zinc deficiency it is helpful to treat the problem with zinc. The maximum daily dosage for this zinc is about 90 mg. The maintenance dose is 50-60 mg. Here, the adage is certainly true that an ounce of prevention is worth a pound of cure.

Garlic is very beneficial. Minced cloves can be added to food, or garlic can be taken as a supplement. A problem with garlic is the odor which can be avoided by using Kyolic garlic or other odor-controlled forms. I recommend Kyolic Formula 104, which has lecithin added to the formula. Garlic balancies cholesterol, prevents high blood pressure and atherosclerosis, reduces infection, and relieves the symptoms of bronchitis and influenza.

D-Ribose sometimes just referred to as ribose is a carbohydrate molecule found naturally in the body that facilitates the production of energy. It is often used by athletes as it aides in overcoming fatigue by helping to rebuild energy stores that have been depleted. This supplement is useful for seniors who sense the need for more energy.

Prostate Support is actually a medicinal supplement having nothing to do with diet but due to the great incidence of BPH (benign prostate hypertrophy) it does affect longevity, so it is included here. These products vary in their ingredients but usually include saw palmetto, beta sitosterol, nettle, pumpkin seed, lycopene, zinc, and a variety of other ingredients. Every man over 45 years of age would be wise to take a prostate support product as a precaution against BPH. However, this insurance is not a guarantee of protection. One problem is that some of these products don't have enough of the most active ingredients in which case the dosage should be increased.

Doctors have long recommended saw palmetto for the prostate, but the most important supplement appears to be beta-sitosterol, which is the active ingredient in saw palmetto. Most beta-sitosterol is derived from saw palmetto and *Phygeum africanum* which are not the best quality. The best source is sugarcane. Many dozens of studies have concluded that beta-sitosterol is the single most effective ingredient to improve urological symptoms and flow.[17] However other ingredients are supportive. Much hype is given to various products, but the test results and practical experience, so far, favor this one ingredient. The minimum dose is 330 mg taken once or twice daily. Keep in mind that hormone balance is important when treating BPH. Beta-sitosterol appears to increase testosterone levels.

Maintaining proper diet, exercise, and fluid intake is very important for prostate health. The Longevity Diet method of choosing foods is very helpful for adequate nourishment. There should be some form of daily exercise even if it's only walking. Sitting for long periods is not conducive to prostate health. If your work requires you to sit for extended periods, get up and walk occasionally. Drinking plenty of fluids is important, but don't drink anything in the last 3 or 4 hours before bedtime to reduce nighttime trips to the bathroom.

BPH can backup or hinder the flow of urine such that it causes a urinary tract infection (UTI). This may be prevented if, at the first sign of a problem, the individual will take either D-Mannose or cranberry extract pills. The cranberry pills are as potent as about 17 glasses of the juice. These products prevent bacteria from clinging to the wall of the bladder. Instead, the bacteria are passed with the urine. If infection occurs, it may be cleared by taking colloidal silver. Mesosilver is the best we have found. This product acts as an antibiotic. Regardless of the fears that have been spread concerning colloidal silver, many users have found it safe to take in doses as large as one tablespoon, four times daily, but only for about five days; then reduce the dosage. If this does not work, you may need to consult a urologist to get an antibiotic.

Due to the prevalence of prostate cancer among men it is important to prevent BPH from progressing to become cancerous. Regular exams and a PSA are important for individuals experiencing these problems. When cancer is discovered, it seems so prevalent that doctors want to cut on a person with expensive surgical procedures or use chemotherapy which is actually just putting poison into your body which harms healthy cells as well as cancerous ones and can destroy your immune system. It is interesting that doctors who would not consider such harsh measures for themselves prescribe it for their patients. There are possible serious side effects to these procedures including death. Be aware that there are many alternative treatments that have been found successful.

One alternative treatment that has been carefully studied and tested by Purdue University is graviola. This product currently costs only about $29.95 per 100 capsule bottle and is said to be 10,000 times more potent than a common chemotherapy drug mostly used for breast cancer. The following testimonial was provided personally to this author.

> "I have personally used the supplement (graviola) for the past four years for prostate cancer. . . I believe that Graviola works faster and has a quality that no other product can claim. It is known to dry up the "pump" that each (cancer) cell has to take in nutrients. When the pump dries up, the cancer cell dries up and dies. . . My PSA has dropped over the years from 6.5 to .5". (Name withheld but available.)

The Rain-Tree product "Graviola Max" may have the broadest spectrum of activity. However, some have reported stomach upset while using pure graviola products. A related product that has also been successful is "N-Tense" which is fifty percent graviola and includes other similarly active ingredients. It is believed that graviola kills one hundred percent of cancerous cells.

Melatonin is a hormone that is not often mentioned, but it deserves more attention. This hormone is currently thought of mostly as a supplement that is helpful to promote good sleep, and it works well for that. In the studies that have been done, men with prostate cancer have been found to have a deficiency of the melatonin hormone. Like many other hormones, melatonin also declines with age.

Roger Mason in his report *The Natural Prostate Cure*, says, "Melatonin's most important benefit is in extending our life span. Lab animals given melatonin in their drinking water lived as much as one third longer. It also boosts the immune system, and may be the most powerful of all known antioxidants. According to new research, melatonin promotes good cardiovascular health, exhibits anti-cancer and cancer-preventive properties and is very important in prostate metabolism."[18]

Melatonin is available in a variety of dosages. It is sometimes combined with theanine, a natural compound found in green tea which provides calming and stress relief. Perhaps the optimal dose is 3 mg. Melatonin is very inexpensive and widely available. It should be taken only at night shortly before bedtime.

What Now? By now the question in your mind is probably, "Do I need to take all of these things?" The answer is, "Yes and no." Of course, you need all of these nutrients, but you may not need to get all of them as supplements. Your individual diet may indicate some of your needs. It would be unwise to take a supplement if you don't need it. There is such a thing as overdoing. It may not be harmful, just not particularly needed. By analyzing your diet or by blood testing and conferring with a nutritionally wise doctor, or a nutritionist, you may be able to determine your need. For example, if you have high blood pressure or if there is a history of heart problems in your family, you would be wise to take CoQ10 and other supplements to bolster your heart.

Simply for the purpose of longevity, which is our main focus, there are a few vitamins and supplements that knowledgeable doctors on aging recommend. These are a multiple vitamin supplemented with B complex, vitamin C, vitamin D3, vitamin E, DHEA, resveratrol, magnesium, and zinc. Beyond that, it will depend upon your individual needs. Having read the information provided, you will understand why these nutrients are believed to be so important and necessary.

Taking so many supplements may seem silly to some people, but do not be intimidated! You are not alone. Your health and longevity are at stake. There are many intelligent individuals, including doctors and nutritionists, who take as much as I have recommended here or more. If all you take were all combined into one pill it may not seem like so much. But that is impossible for, at least two reasons. We all have differing needs, and you cannot get the amounts needed in one pill (think horse pill). When planning your regimen beware of duplications of a single nutrient in various formulations. However, there are some combinations available that are adequate for many people and are less expensive than buying everything as individual supplements. One such combination is *Life Extension's Super Booster.* You would do well to look for those combinations that may provide some of your needs. Of course, the reason for a multiple vitamin is to get a basic combination of ingredients needed by most people, but one pill cannot contain all that an individual may need, so it is necessary to supplement that to get all that you need.

The Overlooked Nutrient

While we give a lot of attention to vitamins, minerals, and supplements there is one vastly important category that we so often seem to overlook. It is enzymes! Perhaps that's because our bodies produce so many enzymes that we are tempted to think that we are okay with that. But, not so!

Especially when our bodies are stressed by illness, injury, or exterior influences, the enzymes that our bodies produce need support from enzymes in the food we eat. That is simply the way we were created. Furthermore, as we age, our bodies lose the ability to produce sufficient amounts of enzymes. It's another effect of aging that we must deal with. Fortunately, we can do this through proper nutrition - again, as our maker intended.

Enzymes are the *spark of life* or we may say they are the *life force* that keeps us going. Enzymes are living proteins that nourish our cells to provide the energy for all of our body functions. Every body system, organ, and cell depends on enzymes. When we ingest food and chew it in the mouth, it mixes with enzymes in our saliva that begin the digestive process. As food progresses through the digestive system, the enzymes are distributed throughout the body. When we feel weakened, our bodily enzymes rejoice at the arrival of reinforcements.

Enzymes are not found in all the food we eat. They are primarily in vegetables and fruits. Although there are enzymes in nuts and seeds, they are blocked by enzyme inhibitors, so that they are not readily available for our use. However, if the nuts or seeds are soaked for a time, the enzymes are released from the inhibitors. For example, we can soak and sprout alfalfa seed to get sprouts that are full of enzymes. Beans should always be soaked overnight (about 10- 12 hours) before cooking to release the inhibitors and also to prevent them from making an individual gaseous when eating them. Just before taking the first bite, a couple of Beano tablets or an enzyme capsule should be swallowed to aid digestion.

Vegetables and fruits should always be eaten raw so that the body benefits from the enzymes they contain. Cooking these at a temperature above 115 degrees kills the enzymes, so the enzymes which had originally been present in canned and frozen foods are killed by the preservation process. An exception is fruit that can be frozen without being blanched. Pasteurized juices and dairy products are also devoid of enzymes. Most prepared foods never had any. Thus we have the reason for eating raw.

This is a very powerful way of eating. In fact, it can actually mean the difference between life and death. Dr. Lorraine Day, who was an orthopedic trauma surgeon and on the faculty of the University of California, San Francisco, testified in her video, You Can't Improve on God [19] that at one time she had a very serious breast cancer. She refused chemotherapy and radiation because she knew how invasive these procedures are. She had tried almost everything else until she was so near death that her caregiver did not know if she would live overnight. Then she started on a raw vegetable and fruit diet and immediately began healing. She was soon back to being her vibrant attractive self. I have read about a lady who had cancer and survived by eating only lettuce. Many people who are enzyme deficient and begin taking enzymes sometimes say that they feel better the very first day and most feel better after only one week. This demonstrates the nearly miraculous power of enzymes.

There are many things that enzymes do for us. Any attack or injury to the body causes inflammation that summons the immune system to respond. It's enzymes that control inflammation and also relieve autoimmune diseases. Thereby they can conquer a dozen diseases. They help to overcome both osteoarthritis and rheumatoid arthritis so that pain goes away. They can lead to incredible improvement in autism. They can help to overcome food allergies and digestive problems in the stomach, intestines and colon. It must also be said that enzymes are a blessing to the heart and circulatory system. They act as natural blood thinners so caution must be exercised by those using prescription blood thinners.

There are seven types of digestive enzymes. They are Amalyase (breaks down starches); Cellulase (breaks down fibers); Lactase (breaks down dairy products); Lipase (breaks down fats); Maltase (breaks down grains); Protease (breaks down proteins) and Sucrase (breaks down sugars). These can be divided into three basic types: amalyases, which digest starches; lipases, which digest fats; and the proteases, which digest proteins. The pancreas is a vital organ that produces most of the digestive enzymes within the body. If the body is deficient in the enzymes that normally would be obtained from food it places stress on this organ. Too much stress on the pancreas could lead to disease, pancreatic failure, and death.

You have a choice of two different ways to get your enzymes. One is to eat as many raw foods as possible. The second is to take enzyme supplements. If you are serious about getting a good supply of enzymes, you may want to use both avenues. If you are taking enzymes to help digest food, particularly cooked food, you will want to take them just prior to a meal. If you are taking enzymes to control inflammation, you would do best by taking them on a nearly empty stomach. Bromelain, which is derived from pineapple, is used mostly for inflammatory purposes on healing minor injuries, for sinusitis, urinary tract infections, BPH, angina, asthma, and rheumatoid arthritis. For digestive purposes an enzyme capsule containing several enzymes is preferred.

One More Thing About Nutrients

When you were studying health or science, you probably learned about **chlorophyll** but then it was largely forgotten because it's not something that we talk about very often. This will serve as a reminder of the importance of chlorophyll in your daily diet.

Chlorophyll is the ingredient in plants that makes them green. The darker green the plant, the more chlorophyll it contains. Powerful animals like horses and oxen depend upon the chlorophyll in the grass and other plants that they consume daily. It is equally important in the human diet for a host of reasons. Chlorophyll has been found to have anti-oxidant, anti-inflammatory, and wound healing properties, but its benefits don't end there. One of its benefits is that it is an aid to strengthening the immune system.

Perhaps the greatest health benefit is because its molecular structure is almost identical to that of human blood except that a principal ingredient in the hemoglobin of human blood is iron and in chlorophyll it is magnesium. Thus, chlorophyll delivers magnesium and helps to transport oxygen to the cells. It is also vital to healthy blood because it catalyzes red blood cells to improve the oxygen supply in the body. A good supply of oxygen boosts the energy level so that a person feels like he has ample vim, vigor, and vitality to get things done. While you may not be as strong as a horse, you get your energy the same way.

Another benefit of chlorophyll is that it protects the body against harmful toxins. It neutralizes and removes air-born pollutants that we breathe. It also chelates and removes heavy metals, like mercury, that gets into our bodies from the fillings in our teeth or from eating fish that contain mercury.

Those who are prone to having kidney stones will benefit from chlorophyll's ability to break down calcium oxalate which is the most prevalent component of stones. Still another important function is that it protects against a host of carcinogens which tend to become more active as we age and some of our defenses tend to weaken.

Chlorophyll functions in the growth and repair of tissue and is even effective in healing infected wounds. For these and other reasons we can realize how vitally important it is to get a good daily supply of chlorophyll to help keep the body effectively functioning.

The best natural source of chlorophyll is dark green leafy vegetables, with spinach being one of the very best. However, chlorophyll is only actively available if the vegetables are eaten raw as cooking will destroy it. Another way to obtain the benefits of chlorophyll is from supplements in liquid, tablet, or capsule form. One of these is chlorella, which is derived from a form of algae. It is also available in products such as Barley Green.

In Part 1 we have attempted to answer the "whys", "wherefores and "therefores" that are the underlying rationale for The Longevity Diet. The reader will undoubtedly want to refer back to the various subjects that have been covered and that is definitely encouraged to obtain a fuller understanding of the rationale for the diet plan. We will now move on to explain the steps of The Longevity Diet in a logical manner to help the reader to understand how he, or she, can succeed in living long and living well.

PART 2
The Steps to Success

Chapter Seven
Step 1: Diet

We have seen that all of the people of the world who live the longest have diets that help them to accomplish this. The dietary plan for The Longevity Diet takes into consideration the best from the various cultures to provide a dietary plan with a high probability for success. This plan is a modified Mediterranean Diet. In some respects it is like a vegan or vegetarian diet, but it has some distinct differences which are made to more appropriately balance the diet and take advantage of the healthiest foods that this world has to offer. When our creator created, He wisely provided all that we need to live long and live well. It is for humankind to recognize this, discover and utilize these healthful foods. The Mediterranean Diet itself has proven to increase longevity and to reduce the risks of obesity, depression, cardiovascular disease, cancer and other ailments that can shorten a lifetime.

But what benefit is there in living long if one cannot also live well? That means that our goal is not only to live long but also to have an alert mind and an agile body; to possess all of our senses including our sense of humor and our sense of the deep meaning of life that was given to us as a birthright by our creator when He made us in His image. By adopting The Longevity Diet, we are learning to live in that image and good nutrition is one of the pathways.

The Longevity Diet focuses on eating mostly fresh raw vegetables and fruit, whole grains, nuts, seeds, legumes, limited dairy products, limited meats (mainly fish and poultry), olive oil, and, for liquid intake, water, green tea (and other teas), and unsweetened juices (fresh preferred).

We emphasize eating raw food as much as possible, although the diet does allow some cooked food, there is plenty of opportunity for enough variety to keep the diet interesting. It must be noted that only by eating raw vegetables and fruit is it possible to get ample nutrients, including the enzymes and the chlorophyll. We have included in this section some meal suggestions and recipes as examples of the variety of healthy nutritious food that is acceptable with this plan.

Vegetables: The daily portion of vegetables is at least three servings. A serving is a half cup. Fresh raw vegetables are preferred because they provide the best nutrition, including all of the enzymes. The best vegetables are the cruciferous ones of the cabbage family. These include cabbage, broccoli, cauliflower, Brussels sprouts, and kale. Dark green leafy vegetables such as spinach, chard and lettuce are also good choices. With perhaps one exception, all vegetables are beneficial and most can be eaten raw. We do urge caution in eating corn. Corn is not a natural food that grows wild anywhere. It was invented by man from grasses perhaps thousands of years ago. Although it is a nutritious food source and is considered as a staple wherever grown, there are two drawbacks to eating corn. The first is that since it is a complete carbohydrate it can be fattening, which is why it is fed to livestock.

The second drawback is even more serious. There are many fungi that grow on corn. Some are actually edible, but one is a significant food safety issue causing serious concern in the agricultural industry. It is called *Aspergillus flavus* and produces a very toxic substance called aflatoxin which is a liver carcinogen. In the U.S. it is currently most prevalent in the South, but it is more common in Africa where there is also a suspected link with the HIV virus. As corn is not an essential food item for any people who are known for longevity we discourage consumption of corn except perhaps very sparingly.

Many vegetables, such as carrots, celery, cucumbers, melons, and some of the cruciferous ones, can easily be enjoyed raw, but others like green beans and peas, are traditionally cooked. Whenever possible, we recommend minimally steaming vegetables over heat just hot enough to boil the water. Potatoes should be used sparingly because of their starch content. They can be baked. The more nutritious sweet potato and yams can also be baked. For green beans, peas and others that need to be cooked a bit, we recommend waterless cooking because that method preserves vitamins that would otherwise leach out from the vegetables into the water in which they are cooked. Waterless cooking pots are available for this type of cooking. When you get onto waterless cooking you will like it. Vegetables with skins such as potatoes, should be washed well but not peeled; many of the nutrients are in or directly under the skin.

Those who have a problem eating raw vegetables because of difficulty chewing them may want to try chopping them in a blender or a food processor. This won't work for salad greens but cole slaw can be made instantly in a powerful blender like the Vita Mix. Carrots and broccoli can likewise be quickly chopped. Using this procedure will make the chewing easier and preserve the availability of all of the wholesome nutrients of the vegetables. Vegetables such as spinach, carrots and broccoli can also be put in a smoothie.

Fruit: Our diet plan calls for, at least, two servings of fruit daily. We have a very large selection of fruits to choose from. Most fruits used to be available fresh only seasonally. Now, thanks to modern transportation systems, we even have exotic fruits like mangos to choose from. Citrus fruit is a great source of vitamin C and should be included whenever possible. Some of the best fruits are those that are commonly grown on U.S. farms and homesteads. We all know that "an apple a day keeps the doctor away". There is a lot of truth in that. Some apple varieties store well and are available long after harvest. A staple fruit of the Hunzas is apricots. They are very sweet and nutritious. The Hunzas dry them for winter use. Most other fruits can also be dried. Fruit like the apricot, prune plums, cherries and many berries can be conveniently frozen. Simply wash, dry, remove the seeds (of stone fruits), freeze and package them. Some fruits like melons are still usually available only seasonally.

Whole Grains: Whole grains are an important source of fiber for our digestive process, so we need at least six servings daily. With adequate fiber we will not be troubled with constipation. Whole grain sources are mainly rice, cereals, granola, bread, whole grain pastas, noodles, and whole grain pancakes. Bread made with white flour is excluded from this diet. If you are a home baker, you may choose from many types of grain to bake delicious breads. In addition to whole wheat, barley, oat, rye, spelt, rice, and teff flours are suggested. You can bake some interesting combinations. Some don't require yeast and can be quickly made. A slice of bread is one serving. A half cup of uncooked oatmeal is a serving and a half cup of uncooked pasta is a serving.

A Word About Wheat: Caution is urged concerning wheat in the diet. Wheat is high in gluten, and many people are gluten intolerant. There are many other people who have intestinal diseases, such as celiac disease, who suffer from consuming wheat. Moreover, doctors have found that the consumption of wheat contributes considerably to obesity. Another concern is that wheat has been found to contain compounds that make it worse than pure sugar for the blood-sugar levels. This is bad news for diabetics. Therefore, while whole grains are a recommended part of this diet plan, we do recommend restricting the consumption of whole wheat. Bake your own bread using the flours suggested that are low in or free of these compounds. Teff flour is particularly useful as a substitute in many recipes. The consumption of wheat is an individual matter, though, so if you do not experience any problems after eating it, you may include it moderately in the diet.

Beans, Legumes, Nuts, and Seeds: Because they are high in protein, beans are a staple item in many diets. Many recipes are available for cooking beans, and everybody seems to have a favorite. For many it is chili or a combination of beans and rice. Beans are good in salads like three bean salad. It's sad that they are considered the poor man's diet; beans are one of the best foods available. They are high in folic acid, magnesium, and copper and are an excellent source of fiber. Black, small red, and kidney beans are the most nutritious and are recommended, along with garbanzo beans. Flatulence is not so much of a problem if they are soaked for 10-12 hours in water with one tablespoon of bicarbonate of soda. Begin soaking by bringing the water to a boil; then cover and let stand. After soaking change the water. Split peas are good when you want something different.

Nuts and seeds should also be a part of the daily diet. They provide fiber, magnesium, vitamin E, phosphorus, potassium, zinc, selenium, and copper, among other things. Almonds and Brazil nuts are the most nutritious nuts, but all nuts are useful. A small handful or about one-fourth cup would be a serving of nuts. Peanut butter and almond butter are included in this category. Choose the type that is natural and does not contain oils or other additives. The favorite seed for this diet is flax seed, which is consumed daily in a smoothie. This seed is a super food because it contains so many nutrients. Nuts and seeds are included in granola bars along with some whole grains and sometimes dried fruit. Shelled nuts should be stored in a sealed jar kept in the refrigerator to preserve freshness. A small handful, about one fourth, cup, would be a serving of nuts, and a granola bar is also one serving.

Dairy Products: Dairy products are a primary source of calcium and protein. They are, however, limited to certain items and should be consumed in moderation. In the diet plan they are limited to the following: non-fat plain yogurt, which should be eaten daily; non-fat or low fat cottage cheese, which may be eaten two times each week; and cheese, which may be consumed as a shredded blend or as dry grated Parmesan cheese in small amounts on salads or other dishes. Parmesan is particularly well suited for more regular use as its total fat is two percent and saturated fat is five percent of that. Cholesterol and sodium are also low in this variety. Occasionally, a slice of cheese may be added to a sandwich. Choose low fat varieties of cheese. Goat cheese should not be eaten due to a potential harmful molecule present in it. Plain non-fat yogurt is the mainstay in dairy products because it contains billions of probiotics which are beneficial flora for maintaining a healthy intestinal tract. Some cottage cheese also has this benefit but to a lesser degree. A serving of yogurt or cottage cheese is approximately one-half cup. Ice cream may be an occasional or rare treat due to the sugar and cream content.

Meat: In the plan of creation, creatures that were intended to be carnivores were created with fangs and claws or beaks and talons. Considering the features of humans, it is obvious that man was created to be a herbivore. The digestive system of humans is also different, making it more difficult for humans to digest meat.

It is well established that eating red meat can lead to heart disease, breast, colon and prostate cancers. You may look at a beef steak and think that it appears to be entirely lean, yet even lean beef contains a good amount of saturated fat and omega-6 fat, which are the dietary causes of high cholesterol. Furthermore, there is a problem because of another substance that is present in red meat.

"Both saturated and omega-6 fats convert to arachidonic acid in the body, whereas the meat itself contains arachidonic acid. One way that the body rids itself of excess arachidonic acid is by producing a dangerous enzyme called *5-lipoxygenase* (5-LOX). New studies now show conclusively that 5-LOX directly stimulates prostate cancer cell proliferation. . . those who do not reduce the production of excessive arachidonic acid metabolites, are setting themselves up for prostate cancer and a host of inflammatory diseases (including atherosclerosis)."[20].

Lead researcher Professor Ajit Varki of the University of California, San Diego, reported on a study conducted there. The study revealed a molecule, Neu5Gc, that is found in all mammals (both wild and domestic) **but not in humans**. It is also not found in fish or birds. By ingesting meat and other substances, humans are subjecting themselves to this foreign molecule. Due to the presence of the molecule, the heart of a pig could not be transplanted to a human as it would surely be rejected. The report stated, "Gradual incorporation into the cells of the body over a lifetime . . . could contribute to the inflammatory processes involved in various diseases." People who eat red meat are at increased risk of having heart attacks, strokes, at least 17 different cancers, diabetes, autoimmune diseases, arthritis and asthma.[21]

> (Author's Note: If this molecule is found in all mammals, **except humans,** it appears to be very strong scientific evidence that man is not descended from apes; rather he is a distinct separate creation.)

Given this powerful evidence of the probable harmful effects of eating red meat The Longevity Diet does not include any meat except fish and poultry, and the white meat of poultry is preferred over the dark meat. However, meat should not be eaten more than one or two times each week. Salmon, trout, halibut, cod, and tuna are the preferred fish. Albacore tuna, touted as the best tuna, should not be eaten because large quantities of mercury have been found in this variety. Even other tuna may have some mercury, so you should not consume it more than once each week. Atlantic salmon is farm-raised salmon that has dye injected into the meat to give it the pink color that ocean salmon has. Use your judgment. Eggs are acceptable on a weekly basis.

For those diehards who choose to disregard the evidence concerning red meat we want to advise you that if you choose to eat red meat it should be eaten infrequently (monthly or less) and should be either oven or pot roasted with low heat to help prevent harmful chemical reactions while cooking. It should not be seared for cooking. It should be slow cooked until very tender. Tenderness aids digestion.

Olive oil: This could not remotely be a Mediterranean Diet without including olive oil since it is of utmost importance to the Mediterranean diet plan. Truly, olive oil is the magic ingredient in Mediterranean style diets that keeps people living long and living well. You will want to incorporate it into your daily diet in as many ways as possible. Many Mediterranean people prepare their food with olive oil and then drizzle more on it before eating.

You will find many uses for olive oil besides putting it in or on your food. It contains omega-3 and omega-6 fatty acids, polyphenols (antioxidants), a good amount of vitamins A, C, E and K, plus many other nutrients, so it has extensive applications for health and healing. It also has cosmetic properties, can be used for housecleaning chores, oil lamps and has even been put in soap.

Extra Virgin Olive Oil is the first pressed and is the highest quality. It should be used as a salad dressing along with either red wine vinegar or balsamic vinegar infused with pomegranate. Use it as a dip for bread and veggies, and include it in the recipes that you cook or bake in place of vegetable oil. Because it has a low smoke point, though, it is not the most suitable oil for frying or sautéing. For these cooking methods, Extra Light Olive Oil is preferred. The smoke point for extra virgin olive oil is 320 degrees F. Always cook with the lowest heat possible and the smoke point will not be such a problem.

Although olive oil contains a lot of fat, it is the most healthy monounsaturated fat and has benefits that far outweigh any negative aspects. You can actually fight fat with fat. Always keep in mind that the body needs some fat to function properly. Therefore, you want to use the healthiest fat and that's olive oil.

Sweets and Sweeteners: Most everybody has a desire for sweets at times, so you will be glad to know that on this diet plan you do not have to deprive yourself totally of the sweet taste; you just need to eliminate regular sugar, to the highest degree possible, from your diet.

Researchers have found that sugar is toxic (poisonous) to the liver. In this regard there is no difference between regular sugar (sucrose) and high fructose corn syrup. Sugar (in quantity) tends to overwork the liver. Consumed as liquid they hit the liver more quickly. Too much sugar arriving at the liver too quickly causes the liver to convert some to fat. This is called insulin resistance. This, in turn, can cause type 2 diabetes, heart disease, and possibly also cancer. These diseases are much less common in cultures that don't use the Western Diet in which more sugar is consumed. Be aware that liver damage is cumulative and liver failure can lead to death.

You can enjoy the sweet taste by using sweeteners that don't contain sugar and have few or no calories and no saturated fat. They also don't have any chemical that can cause the unhealthy reaction which is possible with some that are currently on the market. Our mainstay is **stevia,** which is made from the leaf of a South American plant. It contains no calories, no fat, no sodium, and only one gram of carbohydrate. It can be purchased in packets containing about one teaspoon, which is sufficient to sweeten a cup of tea or in larger packages. It can also be used in some cooking applications.

Another acceptable sweetener is **PureLo LoHan** derived from a Chinese fruit called monk fruit. It is low-calorie and can be up to 200 times sweeter than sugar, so it must be used sparingly. Like stevia it can be used to sweeten your tea and also for cooking and baking.

Still another is **Organic Date Sugar** which can be substituted in recipes requiring brown sugar. It has 30 calories per serving, no fat or sodium and only three percent of the daily value for carbohydrate and fiber.

There are two measures that are used to determine the glycemic value of sweeteners. The first is its glycemic index and the second is its glycemic load. The glycemic index indicates how quickly carbohydrates turn into sugar and glycemic load indicates the amount of sugar that a sweetener contains. A glycemic load over 20 should be considered high. Both measures must be high to say that a sweetener or food is glycemic. Those who are pre-diabetic, diabetic or who have celiac problems will find these measures to be important.

Honey is a sweetener used much by the pioneers before sugar was available. Honey has 64 calories per tablespoon, and it has a debated glycemic index of 55-83, which means that its sugars, fructose and glucose, are rather quickly absorbed into the bloodstream. Medium GI foods have an index between 56 and 69. The glycemic load of honey, which is 30, is also a bit high, indicating that it should be used moderately. It is preferable to regular sugar, though, and unlike regular sugar (sucrose) it certainly is not empty calories. In addition to vitamin C and some of the B vitamins, it provides healthy amounts of calcium, iron, magnesium, potassium, zinc, copper, manganese, and selenium. Additionally, honey has no fat. Some authorities say that a person could consume up to 10 teaspoons per day without being excessive. Because it is sweeter than sugar, most users are not likely to use that much, so it can be considered safe to use.

There are many benefits in honey that justify its use. Pure raw honey provides the best benefits. The consistency of honey depends upon what the bees were feeding upon. Clover honey is most common, but buckwheat honey is also very good. Honey is an excellent source of carbohydrates that provides strength and energy to our bodies. A teaspoon of honey dissolved in tea provides a good morning boost. The glucose in honey is absorbed quickly to give an immediate boost while the fructose provides sustained energy. Honey tends to keep blood sugar levels more constant than other sugars.

Honey has antioxidant and anti-bacterial properties that boost the immune system. While it is not a cancer cure it has been shown to prevent cancer, especially colon cancer. It has been used with lemon, vinegar or cinnamon for a wide variety of home cures. Perhaps most notably, honey is used as a soother for sore throats, and singers like to have some before a performance. Buckwheat honey is useful to cure coughs and respiratory problems. It has healing properties that make it useful for healing wounds including burns. So the next time you get a burn, after running cold water on it, apply some honey.

If your honey crystallizes put it in a pan of hot water for a few minutes. Do not put it in a microwave because this alters the molecular structure of the honey. A Google search will yield much information about the uses and benefits of honey. A word of caution that must be heeded is that while honey has many benefits for older children and adults, it <u>must not be given to infants.</u>

A liquid sweetener that is preferred is **organic blue agave.** This is a natural sweetener that has been around for thousands of years but has not been widely known and used. It has 60 calories per tablespoon, a glycemic index of 15, and a glycemic load of 6.24, which makes it an ideal sweetener. It is 25% sweeter than sugar, so you would use less. In recipes calling for one cup of sugar, you would use three-fourths cup of agave. It has a mild, sweet taste, so it is appropriate as a multipurpose sweetener.

Maple syrup is another natural sweetener with balanced sugars that contains no fat; has only about 18 calories per teaspoon, and has good amounts of calcium, potassium, magnesium, and zinc. It can be substituted for sugar in recipes, with three-fourths cup of syrup replacing each one cup of sugar. Reduce liquids by three tablespoons. When purchasing maple syrup, it is best to get it in glass bottles.

Not more than once each week, you can treat yourself to one modest piece of pie, cake, or similar bakery item. Choose a diabetic recipe when possible or one in which the sugar is substituted. As most candy has regular sugar, it should be avoided; however, there are some diabetic candies that are acceptable. Chocoholics will be glad to know that chocolate is not forbidden, but it must be the right kind of chocolate. It must be dark chocolate that is unsweetened. Dark chocolate cocoa powder can be used to make hot chocolate using stevia as a sweetener. Avoid hot chocolate mixes that have sugar or other additives. Chocolate has flavonoids that assist circulation to the brain and is a preventive for strokes. It also produces nitric oxide, which relaxes the arteries, thus tending to lower blood pressure. Acceptable amounts are one or two cups of cocoa or two small squares of chocolate each day.

Spreads: Butter is high in saturated fat, so I prefer not to use it. I also avoid most margarine and butter substitutes. However, I have found one that appears to be a healthy substitute. It is Original Smart Balance. It is useful as a spread and for cooking and baking. It has good amounts of omega-3 ALA and vitamin D. It contains no cholesterol or unhealthy fats. However, there is total fat of fourteen percent of which thirteen percent is saturated fat, which, everything considered, is reasonable since you will probably not use a large quantity of it. This company also makes excellent mayonnaise dressings; Smart Beat has no fat, and Smart Balance Omega is a light dressing. Other acceptable spreads are natural peanut butter (no salt, oil or other ingredients added) and natural almond butter with no additives. Jams and jelly should be the sugar free variety.

Liquid Intake: It is very important to keep your body hydrated to flush out toxins, bacteria, and any other waste products. Therefore, you should have a goal of drinking at least 80 ounces of water and other liquids each day. Included in this quota are tea and a smoothie in addition to water. Some coffee is an allowable option for moderate consumption, but sodas and other sweetened or caffeine drinks should be avoided.

Green tea and white tea are especially preferred for consumption by those on The Longevity Diet. The reason for this is its catechin polyphenols, particularly one called EGCG which is a powerful antioxidant. It can inhibit and even kill cancer cells without harming healthy cells. It can inhibit blood clots which affect heart health. Some researchers claim that the ECGC catechin is perhaps two times more powerful than resveratrol. Other researchers have found that those who daily drank only two or more cups of green tea suffered fifty-four percent less cognitive decline. It is for reasons such as these, along with green tea's ability to assist weight loss by boosting resting metabolism that we strongly prefer drinking green tea.

That said, there are now strong reasons to advocate also drinking white tea. The catechins in white tea have such great antioxidant power that they are called super-antioxidants. Human aging is said to be positively linked to this powerful antioxidant activity. We just cannot get too many antioxidants! Coffee drinkers take note – coffee falls behind the health benefits of tea!

It gets better still. These teas also have antibacterial and antiviral properties and likely also anti-inflammatory properties. White tea has been called the tea of emperors; it is considered to be the very best of teas. In ancient times, it was indeed preferred by emperors. Its flavor is so mild that you likely will not want to sweeten it.

Interestingly, green tea, white tea and black tea all come from the same plant. The difference is in the time when it is harvested and the way it is processed. White tea is the earliest, most tender leaves to be harvested, which is why it is so delightful. Green tea is the next to be harvested, and black tea is last. They are also processed differently.

This explains why we prefer green and white tea. However, black tea also has its values. Although its antioxidant power is not as great as that of green or white tea, it does have anti-inflammatory ability. You should drink at least five cups of tea daily. Now, if that seems to be too much and doesn't leave much room for variety in your liquid intake, there is a saving grace. Green tea extract capsules are available. Each 500 mg capsule is equivalent to drinking about four cups of tea. It is suggested that you take two capsules daily with a cup of tea. Thus, you get plenty of benefits and have room for more variety in your liquid intake. Still, drink all the tea that you can, and don't overlook drinking plenty of **purified** water.

What about coffee? There is an ongoing great debate about the possible benefits of drinking coffee. While it is recognized that it is high in antioxidants and can do some good things for those who drink it, there are also some major undesirable results. Perhaps the greatest of these is that it causes high blood pressure. The more frequently you drink it, the greater the problem. It can also cause nervousness and insomnia. That it is addictive is demonstrated in those who drink it all week to stay alert while at work and experience withdrawal headaches, drowsiness, brain fog, and fatigue on the weekend if they are not getting their coffee fix. When you want to enjoy your weekend, withdrawal is not a happy place to be! The bottom line is that caffeine is a drug and not an essential nutrient. Those who follow The Longevity Diet will get all of the benefits they could get from coffee without the drawbacks.

Dr. David G. Williams, writing in Alternatives, says, "Consuming caffeine along with carbohydrate-containing foods can double the increase in blood sugar levels, compared to consuming the carbohydrate in foods alone."[22] He quotes Dr. James Lane of Duke University who has done studies on glucose metabolism to substantiate this. Drinking coffee after meals causes a considerable sugar spike.

Caffeine continues to be the leading mental energy ingredient in energy boosting drinks. Dr. Williams says that one or two cups of coffee daily may not be too harmful. The problem arises with the chronic overuse of caffeine in general it interferes with the functioning of adrenaline in the body. "When you block adenosine with caffeine, you're overriding a 'safety switch' that is in place to allow your body the time to repair and rebuild itself."[23] He warns that coffee drinkers should keep in mind that when caffeine is abused, it's like "whipping a dead horse".

Drinking more and more coffee weakens the adrenal glands until they are unable to perform their duties

Other recent research revealed by Life Extension[24] claims that "coffee is the greatest source of antioxidants in the American diet." A considerable number of studies have indicated the potential for coffee substantially to reduce the risk of many chronic diseases. Among these are cancer, diabetes, cardiovascular disease, and Alzheimer's disease.

The many studies involved in the great debate about coffee indicate that it has both its benefits and its drawbacks. Unfortunately, the greatest benefits are not provided by conventional coffees. The greatest benefits have been found in a special polyphenol-retaining decaffeinated coffee that yields a significant amount of chlorogenic acid. The disease-preventing power of coffee is attributed to this acid. A special roasting process has been developed to roast organic Arabica coffee beans to produce this acid. Life Extension is currently the only known source of this coffee. Other coffees apparently do yield some benefits for those who can tolerate drinking coffee. Those who desire to drink coffee should take into consideration all of the information presented here. Coffee is not our preferred beverage, but for those who seek the benefits of coffee we suggest limiting to a moderate intake of not more than two cups daily.

Juice: Drinking fruit and vegetable juices can be very beneficial. Juices purchased commercially are usually pasteurized, though, so all of the enzymes are killed. Therefore, whenever possible, it is best to use a juicer to make your own juice at home. This method does require a large volume of vegetables or fruit to make a glassful of juice, but there are times when it can be valuable to treat certain problems. This author once used carrot juice to treat a stubborn urinary tract infection. It took a lot of carrots, and my skin turned yellowish because I drank so much, but it was not harmful, and it worked! Other juicers tell similar stories about treating an ailment by drinking a juice or juice combination. In the 1950's, Dr. Garrett Cheney at the University of California discovered vitamin U (which is not really a vitamin) as a powerful healer for digestive ulcers. Fresh cabbage juice is the source of this ingredient. About one and one-half ounces four times daily is sufficient. Juices can be made and stored in the refrigerator for a short time. There is literature available to guide you if you are interested in juicing. Juice definitely contains the life force of the fruits and vegetables from which it is made.

You may be wondering about milk. This is not approved for various reasons that we will not elaborate upon here. Suffice it to say that it is not generally suitable for The Longevity Diet. If you want to know more about this, go on the web and google "the problems with milk". Rice milk is suggested as a substitute in food preparation. Organic rice milk that is nutritionally fortified is available. Howbeit, there are applications where rice milk will not suffice. For those few food preparation applications we recommend keeping some organic powdered milk on hand.

Caution: Soymilk has been highly advocated by its producers and has enjoyed some popularity. However, it is known to boost estrogen levels, which can be particularly troublesome for men. Therefore, it is suggested that men, in particular, avoid soymilk. We have noted soy is an important item in the Japanese diet, but not soymilk. Many studies have been done on this subject, the conclusions of which appear to be entirely dependent upon the vested interests of the sponsors especially when they are industry backed.

Seasonings: Seasonings are added to food to make it more palatable. There are also some other benefits, mostly medicinal, for using some seasonings. Most all spices are useful in food preparation. Only a few that are, or are not, most appropriate for The Longevity Diet are mentioned here. Feel free to consult an herbalist or literature on the subject if you are interested in learning more.

Salt: Adding salt of any kind to food is discouraged as salt greatly increases water retention, so it obstructs efforts to lose weight. The other problem is that salt can contribute to high blood pressure. Salt occurs naturally in many foods, so you should not need to add salt to food to get the amount the body **requires.** Salting food is a personal preference, but it is a bad habit to cultivate. Salt is added to many prepared foods and is a good reason for avoiding them. If you are not salt-sensitive, a little sea salt may be o.k., but the product called No Salt is better. There are other ways to season your food that make it just as tasty.

Turmeric: The active ingredient in turmeric is curcumin. It is a strong antioxidant and reduces inflammation by lowering histamine levels. It also supports the liver by reducing toxicity, and it helps to prevent blood clots. It relieves some osteoarthritis in joints. Try adding a little on your salad to add color and derive these benefits. You will find many more uses for this spice.

Curry: This is a mixture of spices which usually contains cumin, coriander, turmeric, ginger, cloves, cayenne, and black pepper. We have already discussed turmeric. Ginger is helpful in relieving indigestion, motion sickness, and morning sickness; 4-6 grams per day may relieve migraine headaches and nausea. Cayenne is a pepper closely related to bell peppers. It is known to help relieve arthritis, the neuropathy of diabetes, and bursitis. Clove oil has been used to treat gingivitis. Some cultures use a lot of curry in cooking and seem particularly fond of curry chicken. Eating such dishes can be both nutritionally and medicinally beneficial.

Cinnamon: This spice is a favorite among many. Not only does it taste good, but it's good for you. Taken daily, it helps weight loss by lowering cholesterol and insulin levels. A daily one-fourth teaspoon of cinnamon can significantly reduce blood sugar levels. Try it on toast or oatmeal. If you eat a small slice of apple pie, be sure it has cinnamon on it.

Garlic: Garlic has been used since biblical times and its usefulness has only increased. It is popular for seasoning food, but it contains a sulfur compound, allicin, that makes it medicinally active. It supports the cardiovascular system, mildly lowers cholesterol and triglyceride levels, is mildly hypertensive, has antioxidant activity, and it aids circulation to the legs to relieve cramping. It also has antibacterial and antifungal properties. Eating garlic regularly reduces the risk of cancers in the digestive tract. A little in your food may not give an offensive odor, but if you want more of its benefits enteric-coated capsules are the answer.

Kirkland Organic No-Salt Seasoning: This is a blend of twenty-one organic spices and ingredients from around the world. It has an excellent flavor that makes it very acceptable for general use.

Things to Avoid

It is important to read labels carefully on the products you are considering buying in supermarkets. Be aware that what a label says may be deceptive, saying one thing but actually meaning another. Don't just accept the words "pure", "natural", "organic", or "low fat" found conspicuously somewhere on the packaging at face value. Look for the Nutrition Facts, which reveal the true ingredients. But then, still be aware that some terms may be a cover-up for the true ingredient, and be aware that government regulations may allow a certain amount of a harmful ingredient to be considered as zero percent, so look closely to discern the truth. I know this makes the shopping trip longer and is a pain, but it's necessary to protect yourself and your family. A little pain now may prevent a lot of pain later.

For example, consider what "pure, natural sugar" may mean. Butter is also pure and natural and loaded with saturated fat. So you can see how terminology can be deceptive. You want to know how much of an ingredient is present in the product. The word "natural" is intended to make you think it is wholesome, but that may not be so. The word "low" may be relevant. Low compared to what?

Here's how to consider some of the label jargon. "Low calorie" means not more than forty calories per serving. "Reduced calorie" means at least but perhaps not more that twenty-five percent less than another product. So when it says "low" or "reduced" you want to know "lower than what?" The original may be so high that even the one marked "low" is not low enough.

"Fat free" does not mean there is no fat. It means that the fat content is not more than 0.5 grams per serving; it may be less, but that is not required. We advise using "fat free yogurt". Does that mean there is absolutely no fat in the yogurt? Certainly not! Reading the fine print, I see that "total fat" is less than 65 grams and saturated fat is less than 20 grams based on a 2,000 calorie diet. However, on the front of the carton, it plainly says "Nonfat Yogurt, 0% Milkfat". Incidentally, the small print on the "Original Style" yogurt says the same thing, and another brand also says the same, so that is the government allowance jargon that all manufacturers use. Looking at the "Nutritional Facts" of the "Original Style" Yogurt container, I see that it says "Total Fat 8g" which is twelve percent of the daily fat value, while the "Saturated Fat is 5g" and "24%" of the daily value. Rather high! The "Fat Free" container's figures indicate zero percent in these fat categories, but still there can be some fat. The point is to study the Nutrition Facts carefully and understand that they may not be accurate.

You will see some things that are said to be "Enriched". The question is "Why"? Why did it need to be enriched? How was it processed so that it needs to be enriched? What synthetic thing may have been used to enrich it? Then somewhat similarly some products are said to be fortified. Fortified products have nutrients added that were never present naturally. Those may include vitamin D, calcium, or some other ingredient. Those words are selling points to make you think it is really good for you. That may or may not be so. Read the label carefully.

When you read a label, you may see some ingredient names that you don't recognize, so here is some help. We have already discussed high fructose corn syrup and how it can be harmful to the liver. It can also lead to diabetes. It is not the same as fructose or corn syrup, either of which is more acceptable. High fructose corn syrup is an altered form of syrup that should be avoided as much as possible. Reading the labels, we find it in bakery products, yogurt, ketchup, tomato sauces, beverages, granola, cereals, and frozen products, so avoiding it entirely is difficult. You can minimize your consumption of it, though. And another thing, you can write to the producers to try to get them to care enough about the people who buy their products urging them to use the most healthy ingredients.

Here are some other things to avoid: products to take it out. That is the best way to effect change.

1. Sodium nitrate and sodium nitrite are found in meat products. They can form several carcinogenic nitrosamines in the body which can cause prostate, breast and stomach cancers.

2. MSG (monosodium glutamate) is found in soups, salad dressings, chips, and crackers. It can be concealed as "natural flavoring", "spices" or "seasonings". This can adversely affect nerve cells causing damage and severe reactions such as headaches.

3. Hydrogenated vegetable oils are harmful trans fats found in microwave popcorn, crackers, cookies, pastry and margarine. They can cause bad LDL cholesterol levels that lead to cardiovascular problems.

4. Aspartame found in diet foods and drinks gets more complaints than any other sweetener. It may cause headaches, memory loss, seizures, and vision loss.

5. Olestra (olean) is a synthetic fat found mostly in potato chips. There are exceedingly numerous reports linking it to a wide variety of health problems.

6. Potassium bromate is a bleaching agent in white flour. Another carcinogen.
7. Food colorings: Blue 1 & 2; Red 3; Green 3; and yellow 6 are used in various candies, baked goods and beverages. They are linked to cancers.
8. BHA and BHT are found in processed food such as potato chips, chewing gum and cereals. They accumulate in the body tissue, causing a cancer risk.
9. Propyl gallate is found in processed meats and is a suspected carcinogen.

As you can see there is a lot of bad stuff out there. If you see something on a label that you don't know about, you should not buy the product until you can learn what that ingredient is. Following The Longevity Diet, you will be using mostly fresh natural products that will be healthy.

Scheduling Your Meals

The traditional way that Americans have planned their mealtimes is to have three meals each day. We call our early morning meal "breakfast", our mid-day meal "lunch", and our evening meal "dinner". We used to call this meal "supper", but the modern preference seems to be to call it "dinner". Dinner has traditionally been the largest meal of the day.

As we have studied other world cultures we have noted some differences and have become aware of some different preferences among Americans. Preferences may be better for health reasons. If you are a working person, you may be locked into the traditional mealtimes, but you still have some options.

Your first option is to adjust the size of your meals. For example, choose a breakfast that is nutritious but not too large. Then, at break time, have a cup of tea or a granola bar. You could have a light lunch and then a reasonable, nutritious dinner.

If you are retired you have more freedom to choose when you have your meals. This is our preferred plan for meals. When you first get up in the morning jump start your day with a cup of green tea. About mid-morning, have a modest brunch. Eat your dinner in late afternoon at about 4:00 P.M. You may later have a very light snack, but don't eat anything for three to four hours before your bedtime. It is not healthy to go to bed with undigested food in your stomach. This causes your digestive system to keep working while your whole body should be resting. Drink plenty of liquids during the day, which will help to control your desire for food, but curtail your intake within three or four hours before your bedtime. This will reduce or eliminate bathroom trips during the night and promote better sleep.

Another option preferred by some is to start the day with early morning tea, followed later with a modest breakfast. At mid-day they have their dinner, which is their largest meal, and have a light supper in early evening. This plan carries them through the day with food in their stomach and reduces their food intake later in the day to prepare for bedtime.

Your choice will be a personal preference, but we suggest that you consider what might be the most healthy and convenient manner for you to plan your food intake. Try to avoid much snacking by increasing your liquid intake.

Meal Plans

Getting a jump start on your day nutritionally by drinking a cup of green tea and continuing to drink it throughout the day is what we call "Drink and Shrink". Drinking green tea will reduce your desire for food other than at meal times. Also, if you are in a sitting (resting) mode during the day, green tea will accelerate your resting metabolism.

Breakfast: Our preferred breakfast is a smoothie made with two or three kinds of fruit, yogurt, and fresh ground flax seed. Add ice cubes and blend it in a powerful blender such as the Vita-Mix. This or a similar blender is highly recommended for preparing food in The Longevity Diet. A very nourishing alternative smoothie, which I refer to as a "green drink", is made with a banana, pineapple chunks, spinach, yogurt and ground flax seed.

Some prefer a more hearty breakfast with more substance. For them, an alternate breakfast is suggested. Some of the ingredients are the same, so both meals provide adequate nutrition. The alternate is a bowl of old-fashioned oatmeal (rolled oats or another whole grain cereal) with the ground flax seed stirred in after cooking. Raisins, Crasins (dried cranberries) or unsweetened apple sauce can be added to the oatmeal (see the recipe in the recipe section). You may add the yogurt to your oatmeal or eat it separately. Complete your breakfast by adding a slice of toast, another piece of fruit, and a cup of green tea. Note: The ground flax is a very important component of breakfast because it is a super food. See the super food section for more details.

Yet another alternative is to supplement the smoothie with toast or a bowl of oatmeal. Some of the smoothie can be poured over the oatmeal.

This breakfast provides the following: two to four fruit servings, one serving of seeds, (with oatmeal, toast, or another cereal) at least one or two servings of whole grains, and one dairy serving. This provides healthy, balanced nutrition to get you going in your day.

Lunch or Supper: Depending upon how you organize your mealtimes, this meal may be mid-day or late afternoon. Following are some suggestions:

Green salad and soup (preferably homemade soup since store bought soups are loaded with salt) or perhaps a bowl of chili or fish chowder. Choose whole grain crackers to eat with soup, and salads.

Raw veggies and a sandwich:

Sandwich ideas: Use whole grain bread for sandwiches; add lettuce and tomato, Reuben, almond butter and jam, tuna salad, chicken, chicken salad, turkey breast, salmon burger, boiled egg, or egg salad. Be creative with your own ideas. Vary your daily choices to avoid too much meat.

Another suggestion is a bowl of oatmeal or other whole grain cereal and a piece of fruit.

Dinner: Whenever you have this meal, it will be the largest meal of the day. It should be a complete meal with a green salad, cooked vegetables, beans and either rice or pasta. You will find some recipes in the recipe section that will provide some ideas. Recipes found in vegetarian cookbooks will generally be acceptable for your meals.

If you include bread in your meal you can dip the bread in olive oil instead of using a spread. Include a cup of green tea with you meals.

Snacking: The greatest failing of those who diet is snacking between meals and in the evening. Snacking is due to an urge to satisfy a pleasurable desire rather than for nutritional need. If your snacking is associated with a particular activity, you may avoid snacking by changing your habits. Keeping your mind busy with reading or another engrossing activity may be helpful. Drinking green tea and water may satisfy the desire, and the liquid intake will be beneficial to you. When you are leaving home, you could take green tea with you in a thermos. Water can be taken in a stainless steel water bottle. Plastic bottles are not safe for water because the plastic contains potentially harmful chemicals that could leach into the water. If you must snack, it is best to eat celery sticks, mini carrots, a piece of fruit, or unsalted nuts.

If snacking is an overwhelming compulsion that you cannot seem to overcome, research has found something to help the problem. Dutch scientists have discovered a gene variant responsible for transporting serotonin, which is a mood regulator in the brain. This mood regulator can cause a person to indulge in emotional eating. The neurochemical process that stimulates this has been found to be similar to that involved in drug addiction. There is no known drug that can control the problem. However, using saffron extract has been found to be a safe way of reducing compulsive eating thus inducing weight loss. It's always best to look for a natural solution for a problem, so think about what you can change to manage the problem. Keep in mind that most any solution will involve willpower and that comes from inner resolve to make a change.

The Benefits of Fasting

If you have never tried fasting you should consider it. Fasting can be done for various reasons, but the most common are religious or for weight loss. If you are fasting for a religious reason, it is accompanied by prayer, usually for a specific reason. Such fasting shows God that you are willing to forgo food (your life source) for a cause. These kinds of fasts may forgo all solid food with only liquid intake (water and perhaps tea and juices). Some do a Daniel fast where they eat only vegetables and fruit as Daniel requested and excelled upon. Of course, that is getting close to the way The Longevity Diet suggests. Caution must be used not to fast too many days in succession since it can cause muscle loss, which is counter to your objective. If you are fasting for a religious reason you don't need a lengthy fast to prove your point to God. After all He is all-wise and all-knowing.

The type of fasting that is our focus here is for health and weight loss. When you fast it helps to remove some of the toxic build-up from your liver, kidneys, and digestive tract. Fasting initiates a process called ketosis. As you fast your body is exhausting your glycogen stores and your liver starts to turn fat into ketones to fuel your brain and body cells.

As has been said there are various ways to fast. Some like to fast for one or more days at a time, perhaps two days fasting and then a day of eating and another day or two of fasting. Some fast only one full day each week, with water as their only intake. One thing about fasting is that it shows you how dependent you are upon habitually eating, perhaps because you have associated it with watching TV, because of boredom, because you are stressed, or even just because. That means that you need to get yourself under control. When you are successful at fasting for 24 hours you will know that you can control that urge. If a person fasts for several days straight the urge to eat will dissipate. That's why some individuals can go on long fasts.

Perhaps you cannot bear the idea of going without food for a whole day. If you have a bad blood sugar imbalance, it could be possible that you couldn't handle it. In that instance, you need to correct that imbalance before trying to fast. You don't want to push it if you have a real medical problem, but you also don't want to give up on fasting unnecessarily. If it's just the thought of not eating that holds you back, that means that: **you are a slave to food!**

"Fasting helps free your mind from the enslavement of thinking you have to eat every few hours. It gives you new options, new freedoms and new self-discipline. It's about much more than simply not eating food for 24 hours; it's also about self-observation and spiritual mindfulness. Why do you think that all the great spiritual figures throughout world history fasted as part of their spiritual practice? They did that because food messes with your head while fasting clears your head. Healthy fasting gives you the opportunity to clear the food-induced cobwebs and see things with improved clarity."[25]

There is an easier and very effective way of fasting for health reasons if it's done right. It is called a "Mini-Fast". For this type of fast, you only need to endure fasting for half of your day, but you need to do it for several days in succession; perhaps five days each week until you reach your goal.

In the mini-fast you would have your green tea, as usual, to jumpstart your day. You would take your vitamins and supplements with your tea. Then you would consume nothing but water or tea until noon, when the fast would end for that day. Green tea helps to dull your appetite. At noon, you would have your smoothie and perhaps either toast or a granola bar, or you could eat a modest lunch; don't try to make up for what you missed by skipping breakfast. You will have your evening dinner as usual.

Now, there is one more very important detail. Exercise is necessary in weight loss to maximally stimulate ketosis. You must exercise during the mini-fast to realize the greatest success. After you have your cup of tea and take your supplements you need to spend 20-45 minutes exercising. It doesn't have to be strenuous; just apply moderate effort. It could be walking at a brisk pace, bicycle riding, walking on a treadmill, riding a stationary bike, using a stair-stepper, weight lifting or a combination of exercises. You could go to a gym or just work-out at home but the exercise is essential to the plan. A few moments of resting during the exercise is appropriate. You will have mostly fasted from the time you went to bed until noon, which would be about 14 hours of your day. For most individuals I think this would be an acceptable means of fasting. When you start seeing the results you will feel gratified.

Recipes

Apricot Smoothie

The smoothie is a very important part of The Longevity Diet and is usually a part of breakfast, except during a mini-fast.

6 oz. Apple juice (unsweetened)
1 whole banana
2 large apricots or 4 small apricots (seeded, fresh or frozen)
½ to ¾ cup plain non-fat yogurt
2-3 Tbs. flax seed (freshly ground)
6 ice cubes

Grind the flax seed in a coffee grinder. Peel the banana and put ingredients in a blender in the order listed above. Run the blender at top speed until well blended. Makes about 20 ounces.

This provides three fruit servings, one serving of seeds and one serving of dairy in a very nutritious blend consisting of vitamins, minerals, enzymes, omega oils, and probiotics.

Smoothies can be made with other ingredients. Almond milk, or Rice milk can be substituted for the apple juice. Always use at least two different fruits. Other fruits that work well are oranges (seedless), pineapple, mango, plums, cherries, strawberries, blueberries and a slice of cantaloupe. A small handful of baby spinach leaves or some broccoli can also be added with the fruit.

Supplements are easier to swallow when taken with a smoothie.

Oatmeal

1 cup of water
½ cup old-fashioned oatmeal (whole rolled oats)
1 tsp. vanilla or maple extract
1 handful of raisins or dried cranberries.

Bring the water to a boil in a small saucepan. Add the oatmeal. After four minutes, add the vanilla. Cook for a total of five minutes. Just before the time is up, add the fruit and then turn off heat. Cover and let stand for one or two minutes to plump the raisins. Can be eaten as is or with a little of a smoothie or some rice milk. Also good topped with applesauce and cinnamon. Oatmeal reduces cholesterol and improves colon health.

Cinnamon Banana Toast

2 large slices of whole grain bread
1 fully ripe banana
Smart Balance spread
Ground Cinnamon (in amount desired)

Toast the bread in a toaster. Remove and spread with Smart Balance while warm. Peel and thinly slice the banana on both slices of bread with a table knife. Press the banana down as if to somewhat spread it. With cinnamon in a shaker shake the desired amount on the banana and it's ready to eat.

Country-Style Flapjacks

Here is a delicious recipe for light pancakes.

¾ cup Whole wheat flour
¼ cup Oat flour (grind whole oats in coffee grinder)
4 pkts. Stevia (4 tsp)
1 cup Rice milk
¼ cup Eggbeaters, Original or Whites, or 2 eggs beaten well
1 Tbs. Baking powder

Steps:

1. Combine dry ingredients.
2. Add rice milk and mix thoroughly.
3. Cook on a griddle with medium-low heat for about 2-3 minutes on each side.

Top with Smart Beat, honey and cinnamon, blueberry syrup, or your favorite spread.

Makes about six, 6" pancakes.

Teff Pancakes

Teff Flour does not contain gluten, so these pancakes are suitable for diabetics and others who cannot tolerate gluten.

1. Combine these ingredients in a large bowl.

2 cups teff flour   2 tsp. allspice

1 Tbs. of baking powder   ½ tsp. sea salt

2. In a separate bowl mix:
   2 Tbs. extra virgin olive oil
   2 ¼ cups unsweetened apple juice (or other preferred juice)
   1 Tbs. pure vanilla

3. Mix the wet and dry ingredients thoroughly.
4. Grease a cast iron griddle or other frying pan with oil.
5. Fry pancakes to a golden brown color.
6. These tasty pancakes can be eaten with or without a topping.

Yummy Carrots

Here's a recipe that everyone likes. It's a potluck favorite.

1-1 ½ lb. of mini carrots
⅓ cup of honey
½ tsp of ground cinnamon
⅛ tsp allspice
1 Tbs Sweet basil

Steam the mini carrots for 18 minutes in a steamer. Heat the honey slightly so it will run freely. Add the spices to the honey and mix well. Put steamed carrots in a serving dish or casserole dish and pour the honey mixture over the carrots. Sprinkle the sweet basil over the carrots and it's ready to serve. Cover and keep warm if not serving immediately. I sometimes omit the allspice from the mix.

Grandpa's Favorite Veggies and Noodles

This recipe features steamed veggies on a bed of noodles covered with spice and cheese.

4-6 pieces per person each of:

Large mini carrots	Mrs. Dash garlic and herb seasoning
Broccoli florets	Shredded mozzarella cheese
Cauliflower	2-3 Tbs Extra virgin olive oil

4 handfuls of whole wheat wide egg noodles (for two people)

Carrots must steam for 16 minutes, depending upon their size, so start them in the steamer first. Put the noodles in a pan of boiling water sufficient to immerse the noodles fully. Cook the noodles for the time recommended on the package (about 10-12 minutes). With 7 minutes remaining of cooking time, add the broccoli and cauliflower to the steamer. Adjust the heat to medium.

Turn off the heat when cooking time has elapsed and allow to sit. Drain the noodles; pour the olive oil over them, and stir to coat them completely. Put noodles on a flat serving dish or create individual servings. Add the steamed veggies. Sprinkle Mrs. Dash somewhat generously on the veggies. Complete by sprinkling the shredded cheese over all. It's a complete meal. Enjoy!

Salad Dressing

1 cup plain no-fat yogurt or Smart Beat or Smart Balance Dressing

½ cup extra virgin olive oil	¼ cup Balsamic or red wine vinegar
½ cup apple juice (unsweetened)	2 pkts Stevia (2 tsps.) or 2 Tbs honey

Thoroughly mix the ingredients together in the order listed with a wire whip. If the resulting mixture is too thick, add apple juice or vinegar to taste. Let stand 15 minutes before serving.

Cabbage Salad

2 cups chopped green cabbage	Shredded Mozzarella or grated
½ cup chopped onion	parmesan cheese
1 cup of broccoli, cauliflower or	Salad dressing (use recipe given
red cabbage chopped	herein or extra virgin olive oil &
Small handful of Craisins	vinegar)

Chop green cabbage and put in the serving dish. Add onion and other vegetables. Cover generously with salad dressing. Sprinkle on the cheese. You may add some turmeric for color and added nutrition.

Gourmet Garden Salad

Dishes like this really make you appreciate a garden for fresh produce. Mesclun lettuce mix is not usually available in markets. Adjust amounts of the following as needed for the number of servings.

Mild Mesclun mix of red and	Green pepper – cut in strips and
green lettuce	chopped
Green onions including some of	Sliced almonds
the green tops	Craisins
Cucumber – cut in quarter strips	Salad dressing – extra virgin olive
and chopped	oil and Balsamic vinegar

Wash the vegetables carefully. Put the lettuce mix in a salad bowl. Add the chopped green onions, cucumber, and green pepper, then mix. Put salad dressing over the mix. Sprinkle cheese on top, then add sliced almonds and Craisins. Add some turmeric if desired.

Spinach Salad

Use desired amounts of the following:

Baby spinach leaves	½ as much green leaf lettuce
Salad dressing – extra virgin olive oil and Balsamic or red wine vinegar	

Wash spinach and lettuce and place in salad bowl, spinach first, then lettuce, then more spinach. Add the salad dressing.

Tuna Salad

Great for sandwiches, on whole grain crackers or lettuce leaves, or plain.

1 can of water-packed tuna – well drained
3 Tbs. of Smart Beat or Smart Balance mayonnaise dressing
2 slices of medium size onion chopped fine (about ¼ inch thick slices)
2 heaping Tbs of dill pickle relish

Mix the ingredients in the order listed. Can be served on lettuce leaves.

Substitute: Baked trout is a delicious substitute for the tuna.

Apple Cole Slaw

A delightfully different slaw.

1 small head of cabbage	4 pkts Stevia
2 carrots of average size	1 tsp nutmeg
1 medium onion	⅓ cup of Smart Beat
1 large red apple (your choice)	1Tbs. apple cider vinegar
1 tsp celery seeds	3 Tbs. Lemon Juice

1. Chop cabbage, carrots, and onion in food processor and put in a large mixing bowl.
2. Mix celery seed, nutmeg, stevia, vinegar and Smart Balance in a separate bowl.
3. Add the dressing to chopped ingredients and stir until blended.
4. Do not peel the apple. Chop by hand into small pieces. Put in a small bowl and sprinkle the lemon juice on it to keep the apple from turning brown. Mix with the slaw.
5. Refrigerate to chill before serving.

Tuna Macaroni

4 cups water
1 cup whole wheat shell macaroni
1 can water packed tuna
2 heaping Tbs of Smart Beat or Smart Balance
2 Tbs extra virgin olive oil
1 tsp Mrs. Dash Garlic and Herb Seasoning
Ketchup as desired

Bring the water to boiling in a 2 qt. pan. Add the macaroni, and cook until tender (about 12 minutes). Drain and stir-in the olive oil. Then add the Smart Beat and the well-drained tuna. Add the seasoning. Serve with ketchup individually if desired. Serves two.

Old Country Potato Salad

Basic Ingredients
4 medium potatoes
4 hard-boiled eggs
1 stalk celery, chopped
¼ cup green onions, chopped

Dressing
4 Tbs Smart Beat Mayo
1 tsp white vinegar
1 Tbs extra virgin olive oil
2 Tbs horseradish mustard
3 Tbs dill pickle relish
1 Tbs minced garlic

1. Wash and boil unpeeled potatoes for 20-25 minutes (until tender).
2. Cube the cooked potatoes (with peels) into a large bowl.
3. Add the chopped eggs, celery and green onions.
4. Pour the dressing over the basic ingredients and mix.

Curly Veggie Noodles and Tuna

4 cups water
2 cups curly veggie noodles
⅓ cup extra virgin olive oil
⅓ cup Smart Beat Mayo dressing
1 Tbs minced garlic
1 can water-packed tuna or salmon (well drained)
Dry grated parmesan cheese
Turmeric

Heat the water in a medium pan to a rolling boil. Add the noodles. When it boils again, reduce the heat to medium and cook until tender (about 16 minutes depending upon the size of noodles). Thoroughly mix the Smart Beat and olive oil with a wire whip and add the garlic to the mix. Drain the cooked noodles; put the pan back on the stove with very low heat and mix in the oil mixture with the tuna. Serve with grated parmesan sprinkled on each serving as desired. Then dash a little turmeric on top.

Crockpot Spanish Rice

3 cups water
2 cups long grain brown rice
½ cup extra virgin olive oil
4 tsp Costco Kirkland Organic
   No-salt Seasoning
½ tsp granulated garlic or powder
2 cups chicken stock or broth

1 cup chopped onions
½ cup green pepper diced
2 cups tomatoes (fresh or frozen)
1 15 oz. can of diced (unseasoned)
   tomatoes
1 6 oz. can tomato paste

Rinse the rice in a strainer and put into the crockpot. Cook on high for two hours, then add all other ingredients and cook another two hours. Fresh or frozen tomatoes from the garden can be used. Hold frozen tomatoes under hot water and skins will slide off easily. Check and add water as needed. (You can speed cooking by slow boiling rice in 3 cups of boiling water on stovetop for 15 minutes. Then start with the boiled rice and water.)

Curry Cauliflower

¼ cup extra virgin olive oil
3 tsp curry powder
2 pkts stevia
1 tsp lemon juice
4 cups cauliflower forrets
⅓ cup slivered almonds

Preheat oven to 400 degrees. Mix oil, curry powder, stevia and lemon juice in large bowl. Add cauliflower; toss to coat. Place in 9x13" inch baking dish and cover with foil. Bake 15 minutes; sprinkle almonds into mix. Bake another 10-15 minutes to get cauliflower slightly brown

Barley Rice Casserole

6 ½ cups water
1 cup long-grain brown rice
1 cup pearl barley
1 14.5 oz can organic diced tomatoes
1 8 oz can tomato sauce (made with no salt added)
⅓ cup extra virgin olive oil
1 Tbs minced garlic
1 Tbs Kirkland Organic No-Salt seasoning
2 tsp Organic basil leaves
⅓ cup shredded cheese (if desired)

Put water in a 3 qt. pan; add barley and rice; cook over medium low heat for 35-40 minutes (The grains should be a little tender). Add all other ingredients except the basil and cheese. Transfer all to a 9" casserole dish. Place in oven pre-heated to 265 degrees and bake for 45 minutes. Remove from oven and sprinkle basil evenly on top. Add cheese if desired.

Fried Green Tomatoes

4 medium tomatoes	1 cup seasoned bread crumbs
2 eggs, well beaten	Smart Beat Buttery spread

Green tomatoes that are light green or barely beginning to ripen are best. Remove any stem and slice the tomatoes, from top to bottom in about ⅛ inch slices. Thin slices cook better. Put the bread crumbs on a small plate. Have the beaten eggs in a cereal bowl. Use a 12" frying pan with a lid. Put about one tablespoon of Smart Balance (approx.) spread in the frying pan and adjust heat to low. Dip each slice of tomato into the egg and then into the crumbs turning over to completely cover the slice with crumbs.

Then place in the frying pan until the pan is full. Cover and cook for about 3 minutes; then remove the lid to turn the slices, then cover again and cook about another 2-3 minutes or until turning golden brown. When done, place the slices on a serving plate; repeat until all are cooked. Add Smart Balance to the frying pan as necessary when frying. Cracker crumbs can be used instead of bread crumbs.

There are usually some small pieces of tomato remaining. Cut them smaller and put into the egg, then add a little chopped onion and pour mixture into the frying pan to make an omelet so that all of the ingredients are used.

Split Pea Soup

3 qts water	1 medium onion, chopped
2 cups dried split peas	1 Tbs minced garlic
1 stalk celery, chopped	2 Tbs extra virgin olive oil
2 carrots, peeled and chopped	

Rinse and soak the split peas overnight. Then add the other ingredients. Heat to boiling, cover and reduce heat to simmer for 4-5 hours. Peas should be tender and the water cooked down. If seasoning is desired use pepper or Kirkland Organic No-Salt Seasoning.

After boiling the mix it can be transferred to a crockpot and cooked on low for 6 hours.

Trout Chowder

If you're tired of eating your trout the same old way try this for a nice change.

2-3 cups baked, deboned trout

1 medium onion, chopped

2 cups boiling water

3 potatoes diced

¼ cup chopped celery

⅓ cup extra light olive oil

¼ cup Smart Balance

⅛ tsp pepper

¼ tsp. sea salt (optional)

4 cups rice milk

2 Tbs flour

1. Sauté onion and celery with olive oil in a 3 qt pan.
2. Add boiling water, seasoning and potatoes. Cook until potatoes are tender.
3. Separately mix 1 Tbs Smart Balance with 2 Tbs flour and 1 cup of milk. Heat to a full boil,stirring continuously.
4. Add remaining Smart Balance and milk.
5. With all ingredients combined heat to a slow boil and remove immediately from heat.

Three Bean Chowder

1 15 oz can red kidney beans

1 15 oz can black-eyed peas

1 15 oz can garbanzo beans

1 28 oz can diced tomatoes

1 15 oz can tomato sauce

1 cup of celery, cut small

1 cup onion, cut in small pieces

1 cup green bell pepper cut in small pieces

2 tsp Mrs. Dash Garlic and Herb Seasoning

Drain the juice from the beans. Put all ingredients in a 6 qt pot in the order listed. When adding the tomato sauce, rinse the can and add the rinsing water to the mix. Bring to a boil then reduce heat to med-low and cook for 30 minutes stirring occasionally. A nice addition is to add shredded cheese when serving and eat with multi-grain soda crackers. This can be made from scratch using one cup of each kind of beans, but the cooking time will be longer.

Idaho Baked Beans

2 cups small red beans
1 20 oz can crushed pineapple, drained
1 cup chopped onion
1 large green pepper, chopped
½ cup honey
6 oz. can tomato paste or 12 oz. can tomato sauce
⅓ cup molasses

1. Wash and cover beans with 2 inches of water; boil for 10 minutes, then soak overnight. In the morning rinse the beans.
2. Put beans and water in a crockpot; add water as necessary; cook 6 hours on low heat.
3. Add other ingredients and cook 2 more hours on low heat.

Three Bean Salad

1 cup small red beans
1 Tbs. Minced garlic
1 cup garbanzo beans
1 Tbs. crushed oregano leaves
2 cups cut green beans or 1 14.5 oz can
1 tsp. sea salt
1 cup chopped onion (red or white preferred)
¼ tsp black pepper
½ cup extra virgin olive oil
1 pkt stevia
⅓ cup balsamic vinegar, pomegranate infused

1. Bring the beans to a boil in separate pots and let soak overnight.
2. Cook the beans separately on a slow boil until just tender (don't overcook).
3. Drain liquid off beans and allow to cool.
4. In a large ceramic or stainless steel bowl mix the olive oil, vinegar, stevia and spices.
5. Add the beans and chopped onion and mix.
6. Refrigerate for at least one hour to cool and allow the flavors to blend.

Hummus – Good for appetizers

1 16 oz can garbanzo beans (or cook equivalent amount of dry beans)
¼ cup of the liquid from the beans
4 Tbs lemon juice
½ tsp. of granulated garlic
2 Tbs extra virgin olive oil

Mash the beans and stir-in the other ingredients. Let stand at least one hour.

This healthy spread is good on crackers.

Vegetarian Chile

2 cups small red dry beans
1 cup pearl barley
1 med-large onion
1 heaping Tbs minced garlic
2 14.5 oz cans diced peeled tomatoes
1 15 oz can tomato sauce
1 tsp chili powder
1 Tbs baking soda

Rinse beans and put in pot covered with two inches of water. Stir in the baking soda. The soda helps to de-gas the beans. Bring to a boil, then turn off heat and let sit overnight (at least 8-10 hours). Drain off the soaking water, rinse and cover the beans with 4 inches of fresh water. Rinse pearl barley and add to the pot. Then add the chopped onion, minced garlic, tomatoes, tomato sauce and chili powder. Cook for one hour or until beans are tender. This can be cooked in a crockpot on high for about four hours.

When serving, I like to sprinkle some shredded cheese on top and eat with multigrain crackers.

If meat is desired, start by browning one pound of ground turkey and putting it into the pot with the beans and barley.

German Cabbage Soup

8 cups cabbage, chopped
3 cups coarsely chopped onions
½ cup Smart Balance Buttery Spread
¼ cup extra virgin olive oil
½ cup flour
4 cups chicken stock (or broth)
4 cups rice milk
2 cups water
Pepper to taste
Parsley flakes (optional)

In a large pot, over low heat, mix buttery spread and olive oil. Blend in flour and add chicken stock and milk. Cook with stirring on medium until it starts to boil. Cook one minute longer, then add cabbage, onions and seasoning. Add water as needed. Cook until the cabbage is tender. This recipe can be cooked in a crockpot. Garnish with parsley flakes when serving.

Onion Soup

This soup is a good way to use extra onions from the garden. It can be frozen for future use. Other vegetables can be added when it's used.

6 cups chopped onions
6 medium-large potatoes
2 qts chicken stock
¼ cup Smart Balance Buttery Spread
¼ cup extra virgin olive oil
3 Tbs Kirkland Organic no-Salt Seasoning

Peel the potatoes and cut into small pieces; cover with water and boil them until soft. Then mash them in the pan with the remaining water and transfer them to the slow cooker. Add chicken stock and chopped onions. Cook two hours on high. Add Smart Balance, oil and seasoning. Cook one more hour.

When using this soup you can add substance to it with carrots, broccoli, peas or mixed vegetables. Cook on low heat. Serve with parmesan or mozzarella cheese.

Broccoli Soup

8 cups broccoli florets and stems, somewhat coarsely chopped but not too small.
3 stalks celery, chopped
1 medium onion, chopped
2 Tbs. minced garlic

3 cups water
3 Tbs. extra virgin olive oil
4 cups chicken stock
1 Tbs. Kirkland Organic No-Salt Seasoning

1. In a large pot lightly sauté the onions and celery in the olive oil over low heat.
2. Add the liquid ingredients to the pot.
3. Add the broccoli, garlic and seasoning to the mix and cook over med-low heat until broccoli is tender.
4. The soup can be used as is or it can be pureed in small batches in a blender.
5. You may serve it with shredded cheese or Velveta Cheese may be added to the pot shortly before taking off the heat. It can be made creamy with a white sauce.

White Sauce

This sauce is very good for making creamed dishes with vegetables, rice, pasta, tuna, for soups and whatever your imagination desires.

1 cup almond milk or rice milk
2 Tbs Smart Balance spread

½ tsp sea salt
1 heaping Tbs white rice flour

Heat the milk in a small sauce pan with the smart balance and the salt. While stirring briskly, slowly add the flour. With medium-low heat, continue to stir the mixture until it thickens and boils for two minutes.

Curry Chicken Breast

4 medium fryer breasts
¼ cup oatmeal
¼ cup whole wheat flour
1 Tbs. honey
4 Tbs. Extra virgin olive oil
1 tsp curry seasoning

Grind the oatmeal in a coffee grinder to make flour. On a small plate, combine it with the whole wheat flour. Mix in the curry seasoning. Hold breasts with a fork. With a basting brush, coat each breast with honey and then olive oil on both sides. Place in the flour mixture to coat each side fully. Place on a baking tray. Sprinkle a little more curry on top of each breast. Bake in pre-heated oven at 400 degrees for about 20-30 minutes, depending upon the size of the breasts. Remove when the breasts are a golden brown color.

This recipe can also be used with fish fillets such as cod.

Sweet Potato Wedges

2 large sweet potatoes or yams
1 ½ Tbs. extra light olive oil
1 pkt. Stevia
1 tsp. chili powder
⅛ tsp. granulated garlic

Wash the sweet potatoes and peel them with a carrot peeler. Cut lengthwise into wedges about ½ inch thick and three inches long. Put the wedges in a plastic bag, then add the other ingredients and toss well. Spread them on a baking sheet and bake in the over pre-heated to 450 degrees for 20 minutes. Stir once while baking. This recipe can also be made with white potatoes.

Breakfast Burritos

3 eggs, scrambled or equivalent in Eggbeaters, Original or Whites
¼ cup finely chopped onion
½ tsp Kirkland Organic Seasoning
1 large tomato, finely chopped or use salsa
1 tsp. basil leaves
4 large whole wheat or multigrain tortillas, warmed
½ cup mozzarella cheese, shredded

1. Spray skillet or grill with nonstick cooking spray; heat to medium.
2. Cook the scrambled eggs in a separate pan while heating the tortillas.
3. Put some egg on each tortilla, and add onion, cheese, tomato or salsa, basil, and seasoning.
4. Fold over the bottom and then wrap the sides and you are ready to enjoy.

Pickled Beets

For the home gardener who is fortunate to have fresh home grown beets.

I quart of beets	4 Pkts or tsp. of stevia
2 cups white cider vinegar	1 tsp of sea salt
I cup water or beet juice from steaming.	2 tsp of allspice

1. Wash the beets and trim the tops and rootlets from them. If the beets are larger than 3 inches in diameter cut off the top and then half or quarter them.
2. Steam the beets until tender, about 20 minutes. Add the juice to the mix.
3. Mix all of the pickling ingredients in a half gallon glass jar.
4. Trim the tops and scrape the skins from the beets. Then drop them into the pickling mixture.
5. The jar can be stored in the refrigerator for fresh eating or proportionately larger amounts can be pickled and processed for later use.

Sweet and Sour Beets

Adapted from an Amish recipe. Beets boost the nitric oxide level in the blood which aids circulation.

4 cups of cooked diced beets	2 tblsp. Smart Balance spread or butter
¼ cup white vinegar	1 tblsp. of blue agave
1 cup of beet water	1 tblsp. brown rice flour

Put the diced beets in a dish. Put beet water, blue agave, vinegar and Smart Balance in a saucepan and heat on the stove. With stirring gradually add the flour to thicken the mixture. Continue stirring until the mixture has boiled for two minutes. Pour the liquid over the beets.

Oatmeal Cookies

⅔ cup of Soft Balance Spread, softened
½ cup organic blue agave
¾ cup almond milk
1 tsp baking soda
¾ cup whole wheat flour (for less gluten use barley flour)
¾ cup Premium Gold all-purpose flour, (gluten free flax and ancient grains)
2 cups old-fashioned rolled oats.
½ cup raisins or Craisins

1. Mix dry ingredients in a large bowl.
2. In a sauce pan, heat the smart balance and milk just enough to melt the Smart Balance. Mix wet ingredients in another bowl.
3. While stirring, slowly add the wet ingredients to the dry ingredients.
4. Drop by heaping tablespoons onto ungreased cookie sheet. Bake in an oven preheated to 375 degrees for approximately 13 minutes.
5. Place baked cookies on a plate to cool. This is a delicious soft cookie.

For variety nuts and/or dark chocolate chips can be added to the cookie mix. The mixture may require some liquid to be added. Use almond milk.

Apple or Pear Crisp

1. Preheat oven to 350 degrees.
2. Thinly slice 4 large apples or pears and put them in a baking dish.
3. Sprinkle on top ½ tsp. cinnamon and a pinch of sea salt.
4. Cover with 1 cup of unsweetened apple or pear juice.
5. For the crisp, mix together:
   1 ½ cups rolled oats
   ½ cup teff flour
   ¼ cup organic blue agave syrup
   ¼ cup extra virgin olive oil
   ½ tsp. cinnamon
   Pinch of sea salt
6. Crumble on top of sliced fruit.
7. Bake 30 minutes for apples (45 minutes for pears) or until the crisp is crunchy but the fruit is soft.

Multigrain Bread

This is a light bread with a nutty flavor.

3 cups hot water
⅓ cup extra virgin olive oil
⅓ cup organic blue agave
2 Tbs. molasses
1 Tbs. sea salt
1 cup ivory teff or barley flour

1cup oat flour; grind whole oats in a coffee grinder.
3 Tbs fresh ground flax seed
4 ½ cups whole wheat flour or
   2 Tbs. quick rise dry active yeast
3 Cups. whole wheat & 1 ½ Cup unbleached all purpose flour

1. Mix liquids, salt and yeast in a mixing bowl and allow to stand for a few minutes for the yeast to begin to activate.
2. Add the teff flour, oat flour and flax into the mix with a mixer to eliminate lumps.
3. Gradually add the wheat flour. As the mix gets thicker you will need to stir with a large spoon. Mix until well blended, but do not over mix. When the mix ceases to stick to the sides of the bowl drop it

on a well-floured counter-top and begin kneading. If the mix sticks to your fingers add a little wheat flour. Knead for about 10 minutes.

4. Have two bread pans or dishes greased. Olive oil or Pam Spray works fine. I use a 9x5 bread dish and a smaller 6 ½ X 6 ½ dish or comparable loaf pan.

5. Separate the dough proportionately; roll and shape it and place in baking dishes.

6. Put the dishes (or pans) in a warm place and allow the dough to rise. Do not hurry this step. It may take two hours or longer to double in size. Caution: Yeast begins to lose its effectiveness if it gets too hot. A room temperature of 75 -80 degrees is good. In winter, I put the rising loaves near the wood stove. Cover the dishes with a towel while the dough rises.

7. When the dough has doubled in size, put the dishes into an oven preheated to 350 degrees and bake for 40 minutes. Depending upon your location you may need to vary the time and temperature for best results.

8. When the bread is baked it will have a hollow sound when you tap on it. Remove from the oven. Coat the top crust lightly with Smart Balance spread or butter to keep the crust soft. Turn loaves out on their sides on a rack or counter-top to cool.

Savory Pizza

This is a delicious soft shell, multigrain pizza.

1 cup warm water	2 Tbs. extra virgin olive oil
2 cups unbleached all-purpose flour	2 tsp. honey or blue agave
1 cup whole wheat flour	1 tsp. sea salt
½ cup teff flour (may substitute barley or another flour)	½ Tbs. quick-rise yeast
	1 tsp. basil

1. Put warm water in a mixing bowl. Add salt, honey and yeast. Mix and let sit for 8-10 minutes for yeast to start working. It will look somewhat foamy.

2. Mix your flours and basil in a separate container such as a large measuring cup.

3. Gradually stir flour mixture into the wet ingredients. If mix is too dry add water sparingly, if too wet, add a little flour. When it gets too heavy to mix begin kneading with your hands on a lightly floured surface or in the bowl if large enough. Knead for about ten minutes.

4. Placing the dough back in the bowl (if removed), coat it lightly with olive oil, cover with a large dish towel and allow to rise for about an hour at room temperature.

5. Put the dough on a lightly floured surface. Sprinkle a little flour on top and stretch into pie shape. Finish shaping with a rolling pin until not more than ¼ inch thick. Then carefully fold the dough and place on baking pan. Any extra dough can be refrigerated for future use.

6. Add topping: First spread tomato sauce evenly; then add a generous layer of pizza blend shredded cheese; follow this with pineapple tidbits, sliced ripe black olives and sprinkle on a little basil or use whatever toppings you may prefer.

7. Have oven pre-heated to 425 degrees and bake the pizza for about 21 -22 minutes, but not more than 25 minutes. Then remove from the oven, slice and enjoy.

Notes on Using the Food Pyramid

Start from the bottom to choose your main dish.

A. Potatoes should not be chosen more than once per week, due to their high carbohydrate content. Sweet Potatoes, or yams, may be consumed as often as desired. Potatoes are best baked or steamed. Steamed potatoes can be mashed if desired.
B. Rice may be chosen two times per week. Brown rice is the best choice; next is Basmati rice. Couscous are high in fiber and can be eaten alone or mixed with rice in equal amounts.
C. Beans could be eaten daily if desired. The most nutritious are the dark varieties; black beans, small red beans and kidney beans.

As most bread has some wheat flour in its content, bread is an optional item. You can bake your own multigrain bread without wheat flour.

When possible, it is best to eat vegetables raw. The cruciferous vegetables are most nutritious; broccoli, cabbage, kale, etc. Broccoli can be included in cole-slaw. Spinach is good mixed into a smoothie. Dark green vegetables such as broccoli, spinach, kale contain the most nutrition. Romaine and leaf lettuce varieties are preferred over iceberg lettuce. A serving is One-half cup.

You may find a variety of ways to include fruit in your diet. It may be eaten separately, included in a smoothie, as a fruit salad, mixed into a rice dish, or with other foods. One-half cup is a serving.

Seeds and nuts can be a snack item or can be mixed into cookies, salads, or other dishes.

Use olive oil liberally in salad dressings and cooked foods. When possible add the olive oil last so no value is lost in cooking.

White varieties of cheese are the best choice. Grated Parmesan may be used as a topping, the same as other grated cheeses. Cheese is a good source of protein, but use it sparingly due to its fat content.

Limit your consumption of fish to not more than two times per week.

Limit poultry to once per week. Eggs may be consumed up to three times per week, either alone or mixed in foods such as pancakes.

The sugar free sweets are the best choice.

Avoid eating red meat, especially beef, except when you are a guest or for a special occasion. Venison has less fat and none of the additives found in domestic meat. Therefore, it may be eaten more frequently than other red meat. A cured venison steak tastes like ham.

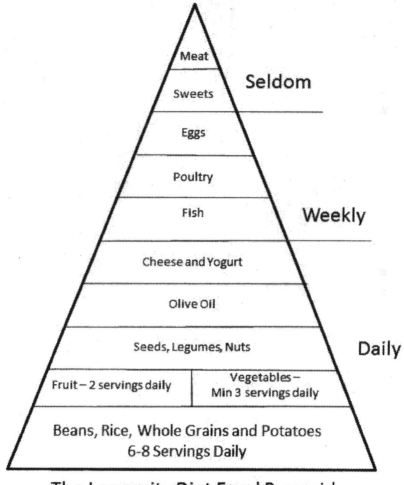

Meat

Sweets

Seldom

Eggs

Poultry

Fish

Weekly

Cheese and Yogurt

Olive Oil

Seeds, Legumes, Nuts

Daily

Fruit – 2 servings daily

Vegetables –
Min 3 servings daily

Beans, Rice, Whole Grains and Potatoes
6-8 Servings Daily

The Longevity Diet Food Pyramid
Use as a guide to meal planning.

Nutrition Facts

Serving Size 1 oz or 1/4 cup (28g)
Servings Per Container 48

Amount Per Serving

Calories 120   Calories from Fat 20

	% Daily Value*
Total Fat 2.5g	**4%**
Saturated Fat 0g	**0%**
Trans Fat 0g	
Cholesterol 0mg	**0%**
Sodium 10mg	**0%**
Total Carbohydrate 21g	**7%**
Dietary Fiber 3g	**12%**
Sugars 0g	
Protein 3g	

Vitamin A 0%	•	Vitamin C 0%	
Calcium 2%	•	Iron 4%	

*Percent Daily Values are based on a 2,000 calorie diet. Your daily values may be higher or lower depending on your calorie needs:

	Calories:	2,000	2,500
Total Fat	Less than	65g	80g
Sat Fat	Less than	20g	25g
Cholesterol	Less than	300mg	300mg
Sodium	Less than	2,400mg	2,400mg
Total Carbohydrate		300g	375g
Dietary Fiber		25g	30g

Calories per gram:
Fat 9   •   Carbohydrate 4   •   Protein 4

PER SERVING:

1200 MG OMEGA-3	170 MG LIGNANS
300 MG OMEGA-6	3 GRAMS FIBER
400 MG OMEGA-9	12 GRAMS WHOLE GRAINS

INGREDIENTS: RICE FLOUR, TCM® GROUND FLAXSEED, QUINOA FLOUR, BUCKWHEAT FLOUR, AMARANTH FLOUR, TAPIOCA FLOUR, ARROWROOT FLOUR, XANTHAN GUM

Premium Gold Flax Products, Inc. (866)-570-1234
After opening store in a cool dry place or refrigerate

① Serving Size

② Amount of Calories

③ Limit these Nutrients

④ Get Enough of these Nutrients

⑤ Percent (%) Daily Value

⑥ Footnote with Daily Values (DVs)

Notes on the Nutrition Label

1. **Serving Size**

This section is the basis for determining number of calories, amount of each nutrient, and %DVs of a food. Use it to compare a serving to how much you actually eat. Serving sizes are given in familiar units, such as cups or pieces, followed by the metric amount, e.g., number of grams.

2. **Amount of Calories**

If you want to manage your weight (lose, gain or maintain), this section is especially helpful. The amount of calories is listed on the left side. The right side shows how many calories in one serving come from fat. The key is to balance how many calories you eat with how many calories your body uses. **Tip:** *Remember that a product that's fat-free isn't necessarily calorie-free.*

3. **Limit These Nutrients**

Eating too much total fat (including saturated fat and trans fat), cholesterol, or sodium may increase your risk of certain chronic diseases, such as heart disease, some cancers, or high blood pressure. The goal is to stay below 100%DV for each of these nutrients per day.

4. **Get Enough of these Nutrients**

Americans often don't get enough dietary fiber, vitamin A, vitamin C, calcium, and iron in their diets. Eating enough of these nutrients may improve your health and help reduce the risk of some diseases and conditions.

5. **Percent (%) Daily Value**

This section tells you whether the nutrients (total fat, sodium, dietary fiber, etc.) in one serving of food contribute a little or a lot to your total daily diet.

The %DVs are based on a 2,000 calorie diet. Each listed nutrient is based on 100% of the recommended amounts for that nutrient. For example, 18% for total fat means that one serving furnishes 18% of the total daily allowance for fat.

6. **Footnote for the Daily Values**

The footnote content may change. Watch for changes.

U.S. Food and Drug Administration, October 2009

Vegetables
Nutrition Facts

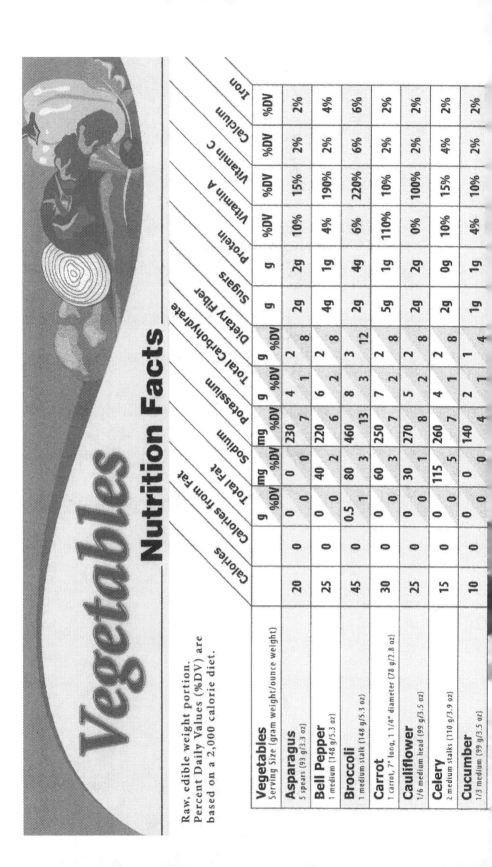

Raw, edible weight portion.
Percent Daily Values (%DV) are
based on a 2,000 calorie diet.

Vegetables Serving Size (gram weight/ounce weight)	Calories	Calories from Fat	Total Fat (g)	%DV	Sodium (mg)	%DV	Potassium (mg)	%DV	Total Carbohydrate (g)	%DV	Dietary Fiber (g)	%DV	Sugars (g)	Protein (g)	Vitamin A %DV	Vitamin C %DV	Calcium %DV	Iron %DV
Asparagus 5 spears (93 g/3.3 oz)	20	0	0	0	0	0	230	7	4	1	2g	8	2g	2g	10%	15%	2%	2%
Bell Pepper 1 medium (148 g/5.3 oz)	25	0	0	0	40	2	220	6	6	2	2g	8	4g	1g	4%	190%	2%	4%
Broccoli 1 medium stalk (148 g/5.3 oz)	45	0	0.5	1	80	3	460	13	8	3	3g	12	2g	4g	6%	220%	6%	6%
Carrot 1 carrot, 7" long, 1 1/4" diameter (78 g/2.8 oz)	30	0	0	0	60	3	250	7	7	2	2g	8	5g	1g	110%	10%	2%	2%
Cauliflower 1/6 medium head (99 g/3.5 oz)	25	0	0	0	30	1	270	8	5	2	2g	8	2g	2g	0%	100%	2%	2%
Celery 2 medium stalks (110 g/3.9 oz)	15	0	0	0	115	5	260	7	4	1	2g	8	2g	0g	10%	15%	4%	2%
Cucumber 1/3 medium (99 g/3.5 oz)	10	0	0	0	0	0	140	4	2	1	1g	4	1g	1g	4%	10%	2%	2%

Vegetable	Calories	Calories from Fat	Total Fat	Sodium	Potassium	Total Carbohydrate	Dietary Fiber	Sugars	Protein	Vitamin A	Vitamin C	Calcium	Iron
Green Onion 1/4 cup chopped (25 g/0.9 oz)	10	0	0g 0%	10mg 0%	70mg 2%	2g 1%	1g 4%	1g	1g	2%	8%	2%	2%
Iceberg Lettuce 1/6 medium head (89 g/3.2 oz)	10	0	0g 0%	10mg 0%	125mg 4%	2g 1%	1g 4%	2g	1g	6%	6%	2%	2%
Leaf Lettuce 1 1/2 cups shredded (85 g/3.0 oz)	15	0	0g 0%	35mg 1%	170mg 5%	2g 1%	1g 4%	1g	1g	130%	6%	2%	4%
Mushrooms 5 medium (84 g/3.0 oz)	20	0	0g 0%	15mg 0%	300mg 9%	3g 1%	1g 4%	0g	3g	0%	2%	0%	2%
Onion 1 medium (148 g/5.3 oz)	45	0	0g 0%	5mg 0%	190mg 5%	11g 4%	3g 12%	9g	1g	0%	20%	4%	4%
Potato 1 medium (148 g/5.3 oz)	110	0	0g 0%	0mg 0%	620mg 18%	26g 9%	2g 8%	1g	3g	0%	45%	2%	6%
Radishes 7 radishes (85 g/3.0 oz)	10	0	0g 0%	55mg 2%	190mg 5%	3g 1%	1g 4%	2g	0g	0%	30%	2%	2%
Summer Squash 1/2 medium (98 g/3.5 oz)	20	0	0g 0%	0mg 0%	260mg 7%	4g 1%	2g 8%	2g	1g	6%	30%	2%	2%
Sweet Corn kernels from 1 medium ear (90 g/3.2 oz)	90	20	2.5g 4%	0mg 0%	250mg 7%	18g 6%	2g 8%	5g	4g	2%	10%	0%	2%
Sweet Potato 1 medium, 5" long, 2"diameter (130 g/4.6 oz)	100	0	0g 0%	70mg 3%	440mg 13%	23g 8%	4g 16%	7g	2g	120%	30%	4%	4%
Tomato 1 medium (148 g/5.3 oz)	25	0	0g 0%	20mg 1%	340mg 10%	5g 2%	1g 4%	3g	1g	20%	40%	2%	4%

Most vegetables provide negligible amounts of saturated fat, *trans* fat, and cholesterol.

U.S. Food and Drug Administration
(January 1, 2008)

Fruits

Nutrition Facts

Raw, edible weight portion. Percent Daily Values (%DV) are based on a 2,000 calorie diet.

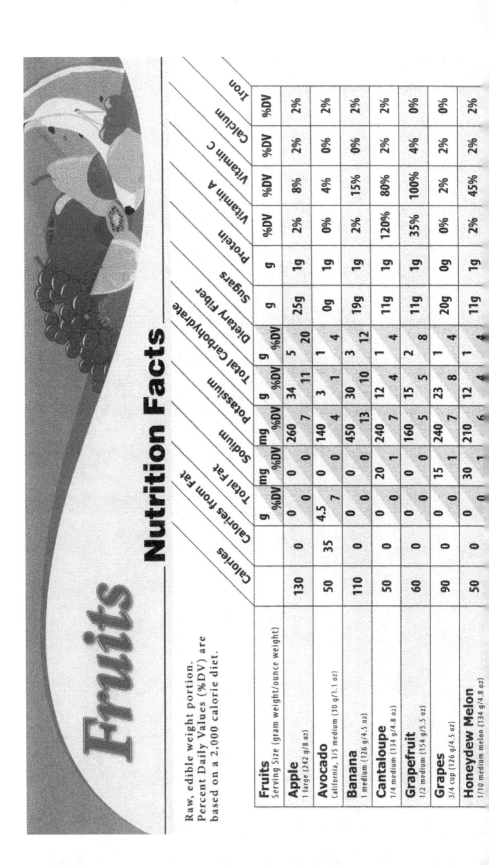

Fruits Serving Size (gram weight/ounce weight)	Calories	Calories from Fat	Total Fat (g)	%DV	Sodium (mg)	%DV	Potassium (mg)	%DV	Total Carbohydrate (g)	%DV	Dietary Fiber (g)	%DV	Sugars (g)	Protein (g)	Vitamin A %DV	Vitamin C %DV	Calcium %DV	Iron %DV
Apple 1 large (242 g/8 oz)	130	0	0	0	0	0	260	7	34	11	5	20	25g	1g	2%	8%	2%	2%
Avocado (california, 1/5 medium (30 g/1.1 oz)	50	35	4.5	7	0	0	140	4	3	1	1	4	0g	1g	0%	4%	0%	2%
Banana 1 medium (126 g/4.5 oz)	110	0	0	0	0	0	450	13	30	10	3	12	19g	1g	2%	15%	0%	2%
Cantaloupe 1/4 medium (134 g/4.8 oz)	50	0	0	0	20	1	240	7	12	4	1	4	11g	1g	120%	80%	2%	2%
Grapefruit 1/2 medium (154 g/5.5 oz)	60	0	0	0	0	0	160	5	15	5	2	8	11g	1g	35%	100%	4%	0%
Grapes 3/4 cup (126 g/4.5 oz)	90	0	0	0	15	1	240	7	23	8	1	4	20g	0g	0%	2%	2%	0%
Honeydew Melon 1/10 medium melon (134 g/4.8 oz)	50	0	0	0	30	1	210	6	12	4	1	4	11g	1g	2%	45%	2%	2%

Fruit (serving)	Calories	Calories from Fat	Total Fat (g)	Sodium (mg)	Potassium (mg)	Potassium %DV	Total Carb. (g)	Carb. %DV	Dietary Fiber (g)	Fiber %DV	Sugars	Protein	Vit. A	Vit. C	Calcium	Iron
Lime 1 medium (67 g/2.4 oz)	20	0	0	0	75	2	7	2	2	8	0g	0g	0%	35%	0%	0%
Nectarine 1 medium (140 g/5.0 oz)	60	5	0.5	1	250	7	15	5	2	8	11g	1g	8%	15%	0%	2%
Orange 1 medium (154 g/5.5 oz)	80	0	0	0	250	7	19	6	3	12	14g	1g	2%	130%	6%	0%
Peach 1 medium (147 g/5.3 oz)	60	0	0.5	1	230	7	15	5	2	8	13g	1g	6%	15%	0%	2%
Pear 1 medium (166 g/5.9 oz)	100	0	0	0	190	5	26	9	6	24	16g	1g	0%	10%	2%	0%
Pineapple 2 slices, 3" diameter, 3/4" thick (112 g/4 oz)	50	0	0	10	120	3	13	4	1	4	10g	1g	2%	50%	2%	2%
Plums 2 medium (151 g/5.4 oz)	70	0	0	0	230	7	19	6	2	8	16g	1g	8%	10%	0%	2%
Strawberries 8 medium (147g/5.3 oz)	50	0	0	0	170	5	11	4	2	8	8g	1g	0%	160%	2%	2%
Sweet Cherries 21 cherries; 1 cup (140 g/5.0 oz)	100	0	0	0	350	10	26	9	1	4	16g	1g	2%	15%	2%	2%
Tangerine 1 medium (109 g/3.9 oz)	50	0	0	0	160	5	13	4	2	8	9g	1g	6%	45%	4%	0%
Watermelon 1/18 medium melon; 2 cups diced pieces (280 g/10.0 oz)	80	0	0	0	270	8	21	7	1	4	20g	1g	30%	25%	2%	4%

Most fruits provide negligible amounts of saturated fat, *trans* fat, and cholesterol; avocados provide 0.5 g of saturated fat per ounce.

U.S. Food and Drug Administration
(January 1, 2008)

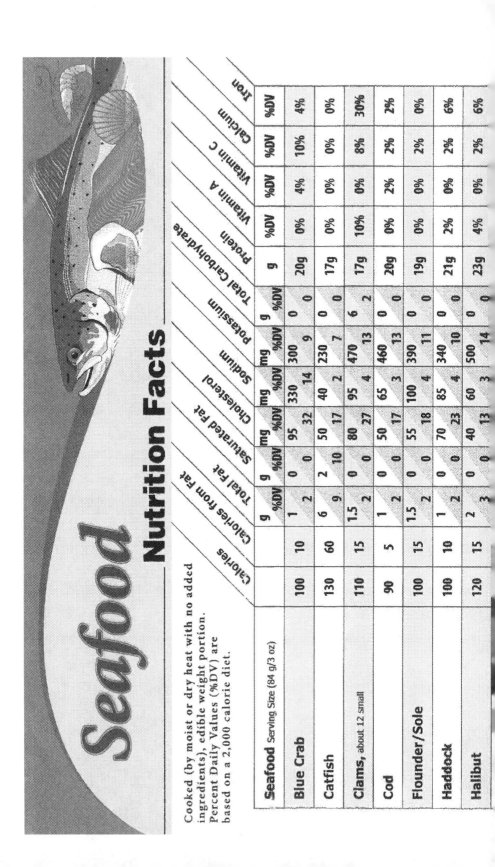

Seafood
Nutrition Facts

Cooked (by moist or dry heat with no added ingredients), edible weight portion. Percent Daily Values (%DV) are based on a 2,000 calorie diet.

Seafood (Serving Size 84 g/3 oz)	Calories	Calories from Fat	Total Fat (g)	Total Fat %DV	Saturated Fat (g)	Sat Fat %DV	Cholesterol (mg)	Chol %DV	Sodium (mg)	Sodium %DV	Potassium (mg)	Potassium %DV	Total Carbohydrate (g)	Carb %DV	Protein (g)	Protein %DV	Vitamin A %DV	Vitamin C %DV	Calcium %DV	Iron %DV
Blue Crab	100	10	1	2	0	0	95	32	330	14	300	9	0	0	20g		0%	4%	10%	4%
Catfish	130	60	6	9	2	10	50	17	40	2	230	7	0	0	17g		0%	0%	0%	0%
Clams, about 12 small	110	15	1.5	2	0	0	80	27	95	4	470	13	6	2	17g		10%	0%	8%	30%
Cod	90	5	1	2	0	0	50	17	65	3	460	13	0	0	20g		0%	2%	2%	2%
Flounder/Sole	100	15	1.5	2	0	0	55	18	100	4	390	11	0	0	19g		0%	0%	2%	0%
Haddock	100	10	1	2	0	0	70	23	85	4	340	10	0	0	21g	2%	2%	0%	2%	6%
Halibut	120	15	2	3	0	0	40	13	60	3	500	14	0	0	23g	4%	4%	0%	2%	6%

Seafood	Calories	Calories from Fat	Total Fat (g)	Total Fat %DV	Saturated Fat (g)	Sat Fat %DV	Cholesterol (mg)	Cholesterol %DV	Sodium (mg)	Sodium %DV	Potassium (mg)	Potassium %DV	Total Carb (g)	Protein	Vitamin A	Vitamin C	Calcium	Iron
Orange Roughy	80	5	1	2	0	0	20	7	70	3	340	10	0	16g	2%	0%	4%	2%
Oysters, about 12 medium	100	35	4	6	1	5	80	27	300	13	220	6	6	10g	0%	6%	6%	45%
Pollock	90	10	1	2	0	0	80	27	110	5	370	11	0	20g	2%	0%	0%	2%
Rainbow Trout	140	50	6	9	2	10	55	18	35	1	370	11	0	20g	4%	4%	8%	2%
Rockfish	110	15	2	3	0	0	40	13	70	3	440	13	0	21g	4%	0%	2%	2%
Salmon, Atlantic/Coho/Sockeye/Chinook	200	90	10	15	2	10	70	23	55	2	430	12	0	24g	4%	4%	2%	2%
Salmon, Chum/Pink	130	40	4	6	1	5	70	23	65	3	420	12	0	22g	2%	0%	2%	4%
Scallops, about 6 large or 14 small	140	10	1	2	0	0	65	22	310	13	430	12	5	27g	2%	0%	4%	14%
Shrimp	100	10	1.5	2	0	0	170	57	240	10	220	6	0	21g	4%	4%	6%	10%
Swordfish	120	50	6	9	1.5	8	40	13	100	4	310	9	0	16g	2%	2%	0%	6%
Tilapia	110	20	2.5	4	1	5	75	25	30	1	360	10	0	22g	0%	2%	0%	2%
Tuna	130	15	1.5	2	0	0	50	17	40	2	480	14	0	26g	2%	2%	2%	4%

Seafood provides negligible amounts of *trans* fat, dietary fiber, and sugars.

U.S. Food and Drug Administration
(January 1, 2008)

Super Foods

Super Foods are foods that are considered to be especially nutritious and beneficial for health and longevity. Good nutrition is the best way to put the brakes on the aging process. There are those who declare certain foods to be best for one reason or another, but they may not be commonly available, or they may be expensive. We are recommending here foods that are usually available and not too costly.

Super foods are usually natural whole foods. With the exception of cheese and yogurt, they are not processed in any way. Processing such as that done to make potato chips destroys any value originally in the food and further degrades it by deep frying in oil and covering with food additives. It is always best, whenever possible to get your nutrition from natural sources. The foods presented here are recommended to be included in The Longevity Diet.

Flax Seed:

This small seed is one of the most nutritional foods to be found. In many ways it is similar to grains due to its content of vitamins and minerals. However, the amount of fiber, antioxidants and particularly omega-3 fatty acids make it especially desirable for daily use in your diet. It is low in carbohydrates, which combined with its high fiber and healthy fats, make it ideal for weight loss and maintenance.

Flax is a rich source of energy and has 32.5% of the daily requirement of protein, but where it shines is in that it also gives you 8g of omega-3 fatty acids. They are a good source of lignans, which are phytoestrogens that have antioxidant and cancer prevention properties.

Flax seeds are particularly high in many essential vitamins and minerals, including vitamin E (19.95mg per gram), Thiamin (1.64 mg), niacin (3.08 mg), vitamin K (4.3 mg). Its minerals include, potassium (813 mg), calcium (255 mg), magnesium (392 mg), Zinc (4.34 mg) and iron 5.73 mg). There are others in lesser amounts.

An additional bonus is that they are high in lutien-zeaxanthin, which is known to retard the progression of macular degeneration.

If you are just getting started eating flax, you should go slow and gradually increase the amount you ingest as it may affect your bowels due to its high fiber content so adding a great deal suddenly may stress your bowels. The seeds should be ground in a coffee grinder for about five seconds. They can be used in smoothies, on cooked oatmeal, on salads, yogurt, or in baking.

Oatmeal:

This is often referred to as rolled oats and is available in two forms. The original rolled oats, sometimes called old-fashioned oatmeal, is the whole grain which we prefer for most uses, but the quick-cooking form, which uses only the heart of the grain, works better for some recipes. The whole grain contains more fiber and nutrients.

The beta glucans in oatmeal are very useful for heart health. Their heart benefit is due to their ability to lower serum cholesterol levels, and oatmeal's high fiber content makes it good for colon health.

Oats are low in calories and high in protein. They are a rich source of magnesium, potassium, copper, zinc, selenium, thiamine, and pantothenic acid. They are a good source of vitamin R (tocotrienols and tocopherols of the vitamin E family). They also contain phytonutrients, including lignans, and protease inhibitors. The combination of nutrients makes oats an excellent food, capable of promoting good health and reducing the possibility of disease states.

Oats should not be thought of only as a breakfast food. They can be a healthy part of any meal. It is used in many recipes for cookies and bread and Oatmeal can also be dressed with fruit which adds to the nutritional value of a meal.

Apricots:

The apricot is believed to have originated in southern China, but due to its delicious sweet taste, it has traveled around the world wherever the climate is suitable for its cultivation. Solomon referred to apricots as "apples of gold". They are so nutritious that they are prized as one of the staple foods of the Hunzas in northern Pakistan. They eat them fresh and dry them in the sun for later use.

Apricots get their sweet flavor from 3.23 grams of sugars which are a combination of sucrose, glucose, and fructose. The fresh apricots are high in fiber, and can have a laxative effect which, of course, prevents constipation and is good for the colon. If a person is accustomed to eating them this is not a problem.

This fruit is a rich source of vitamin A (674 IU) and beta carotene (383 mcg), which converts to vitamin A. Because they also contain 31 mcg of lutein- zeaxanthin, they are very good for the eyes. Beta carotene also helps to prevent heart disease, which explains why the Hunzas have little difficulty with that.

They are high in potassium (91 mg), vitamin C (3.5 mg), folate (3 mg), and vitamin K (1.2 mg), as well as numerous other nutrients in smaller amounts. The high nutritive value of apricots helps to prevent and remove gallstones, intestinal worms and aids in digestion since it reacts as an alkaline to break down food particles. As it has cosmetic value it is used in facial scrubs and other cosmetics.

Apricots are a soft fruit so they are difficult to preserve by canning when they are ripe, so the best methods of preserving them are by drying or freezing them. Freezing is simply a matter of washing the apricots, cutting out the pits, laying them out to evaporate excess moisture and then bagging them in plastic freezer bags. The dried fruit can be eaten as is, while the frozen fruit can be eaten when barely thawed, or used in smoothies or other recipes.

Bananas:

Some diet plans don't recommend eating bananas because the average banana has 100 calories. However, we do include them because they have so many benefits that outweigh the calorie load. But we advise limited consumption of not more than one or two per day unless you make a calorie trade-off. Bananas are most famous for their great amount of potassium (467.28 mg) which is good for regulating blood pressure and combined with the ease of digesting them, they can help to settle an upset stomach or soothe a stomach ulcer. It also goes a long way in preventing leg cramps following strenuous exercise.

Bananas are a good source of prebiotics, so called because they nourish friendly probiotic bacteria in the colon during the digestive process. These bacterias produce digestive enzymes that improve the ability to absorb nutrients and control harmful bacteria.

Bananas provide 30 grams of carbohydrates, which fuel the body's needs for muscle and central nervous system activity. Although they are high in calories, they are also high in soluble fiber that breaks down slowly during digestion and prolongs the expenditure of energy. This is also helpful to the dieter because the feeling of fullness remains longer.

This nutrient-rich food contains natural sugars that give a quick boost when eaten, but it's fat-free, so the calories don't tend to stay with you. An added benefit of bananas is that they contain mood-regulating tryptophan, which helps to boost serotonin levels. They also contain B vitamins, which also creates serotonin. So eating bananas may help to keep you in a good mood.

You should enjoy a banana each day in your smoothie. Their mild flavor blends well with those of the other ingredients that you use. To get the full benefit of nutrients, bananas should be eaten when they are fully ripe. Although they may appear somewhat brown on the outside, the fruit is fine, unless they are truly overripe. While most people enjoy eating bananas, there are some who, regretfully, are allergic to them.

Blueberries:

Nearly all berries, including grapes and cherries, are very high in nutritional value, particularly in antioxidants. In laboratory studies extracts of various commonly eaten berries demonstrated the ability to kill, oral, breast and prostate cancer cells.

The very high antioxidant capacity of blueberries has been shown to be particularly helpful in combating the aging effects of oxidative stress that occurs when insufficient supplies of blood and oxygen reach the human brain. Of 20 different fruits tested by the United States Department of Agriculture for antioxidant levels, blueberries were No. 1 in antioxidants. The polyphenols in blueberries help to control inflammations in the brain and are also believed to aid age-related nerve cell functioning.

As people age there is a natural tendency for the body to decline in its ability to protect itself from oxidative damage and inflammation. There are compounds called polyphenols in foods such as fruits, vegetables, and nuts that have an antioxidant and anti-inflammatory ability that protects consumers from this decline.

Shibu Poulose of the US Department of Agriculture Human Nutrition Research Center in Boston reported to the 240th National meeting of the American Chemical Society, "Our research suggests that the polyphenolics in berries have a rescuing effect. They seem to restore the normal housekeeping function." This indicates the possibility of restoring lost abilities by eating berries.

If you live where you can obtain wild blueberries, you are most fortunate because wild blueberries, due to their deep blue-purple pigments, have been found to have 48% more antioxidants and anti-inflammatory capabilities than cultivated blueberries.

Blueberries have also been found to protect against diabetes and urinary tract problems. Similar to cranberry juice or extract, they prevent bacteria from adhering to the wall of the bladder, consequently passing them out with the urine instead.

These berries are especially high in vitamin A (79.9 IU), folate (8.9 mcg), potassium (114 mg), phosphorous (17.8 mg), calcium (8.9 mg), magnesium (8.9 mg) and lutein +zeaxanthin (118 mg) which makes them very eye healthy.

There are many uses for blueberries including eating fresh, putting them in your smoothie or in pancakes, or add them to your cereal. Although some like to put them in baked foods, keep in mind that heat above 115 degrees kills the enzymes in foods. If they are not going to be consumed immediately, they should be in a closed container kept in the refrigerator. They will keep better if they are not washed until just before they are to be eaten.

Cranberries:

These berries, closely related to the blueberry, are enjoyed as a colorful addition to a holiday meal. However, the principle benefit of eating cranberries is the prevention of urinary tract problems. This is largely due to the high level of antioxidants found in these berries.

Although the helpful benefits of drinking cranberry juice have been known for many years it was not understood why. Researchers now believe that the berries contain properties that prevent bacteria (*Escherichia coli*) from adhering to the wall of the bladder and to the urethra where they can propagate and cause infection.

Cranberries have also been found useful for sufferers of peptic ulcers. Researchers are now conducting studies to determine the possible benefits to those who have cancers or are at risk for atherosclerosis.

Cranberries provide a good energy boost with 18% of the daily energy value. They are also high in vitamins C and K and manganese. They are available in canned sauces the year around as well as in juice. As they are tart, the juice is often mixed with other juices such as apple or raspberry. Check the label to be sure that no sugar is added. The best form for those wanting protection from urinary problems is capsules containing the extract. One of these is equal to about 17 glasses of juice, which makes it very cost effective.

Broccoli:

Some of the most nutritionally valuable vegetables are those of the cruciferous family, which includes cabbage, broccoli, cauliflower, and Brussels sprouts. The star among these is broccoli as it is very high in many vitamins and minerals while containing only 31 calories in one cupful. The same amount of raw broccoli contains 561 IU of vitamin A, 81.2 mg of vitamin C, 92.5 mg of vitamin K, 57.3 mg of folate, 42.8 mg calcium, 206 mg of potassium, 60.1 mg of phosperous, 2.3 mg of selenium, and a whopping 1,277 mg of lutein and zeaxanthin . It also has a good amount of fiber and protein.

The most outstanding thing about broccoli is its phytochemical compounds that make it a potent defense against colon, breast, prostate, cervical, and other cancers. It inhibits angiogenesis, thus preventing the ability of a tumor to supply itself with blood, potentially causing the death of the cancerous cell.

In addition to its cancer fighting ability, broccoli is also helpful in producing enzymes that detoxify the liver.

To derive the benefits of broccoli it is best to eat it raw or only lightly steamed to preserve its enzymes. Many people who dislike the taste of broccoli alone like it with cheese. Try it raw dipped in melted cheese, and you likely will find it tasty.

Spinach:

Of the green leafy vegetables, spinach provides the most complete nutrition. A one cup serving of spinach contains 2813 IU of vitamin A, 1688mcg of beta carotene, 8.4 mg of vitamin C, 145 mcg of vitamin K, 58.2 mcg of folate, 5.4 mg of choline, 165 mg of betaine, and 3659 mcg of lutein-zeaxanthin. It also contains Omega-3 (41.4 mg) and Omega-6 (7.8 mg). Due to its dark green color, it is loaded with chlorophyll. You could not ask for a healthier vegetable.

With all of these nutrients in these proportions and many more in lesser amounts it is understandable that its nutrient balance score is 91 out of a possible 100 and its amino acid score is over the top at 119 out of a possible 100. Actually the only drawback to eating spinach is that it is one of the vegetables with the highest amount of pesticide contamination, so it is very important to buy organic unless you are blessed to raise your own.

Baby spinach seems to be the most popular because it is very tender. It is tasty in salads and can be put in sandwiches instead of lettuce. It can also be added to a smoothie. All varieties of spinach are similar in nutritional value.

Individuals on a weight loss program love spinach because it has only 6.9 calories in a one cup serving, so there is little concern about how much you eat. It is always best to eat spinach as fresh as possible because it loses nutrients as it gets older and begins to wilt.

Cucumbers:

This humble vegetable gains our respect when we realize all of its powerful properties. Its nutritional content is only part of the story. For each 100 grams of cucumber consumed it delivers 147 mg of potassium which helps to reduce blood pressure. It has 105 IU of vitamin A, and 2.3 mg of vitamin C. There is 24 mg of phosphorous (which aids the nervous system and promotes emotional stability), and 16.4 mcg of vitamin K, which controls blood clotting and increases bone mass. It also has 23 mcg of lutein-zeaxanthin which helps to prevent macular degeneration. Cucumbers are a good source of fiber and have only 15 calories per serving, so they are ideal for a low calorie diet.

Cucumbers have a mild diuretic property due to the large amount of water they contain. They are also an aid in instances of liver, bladder, kidney and pancreatic disease. They contain an enzyme that aids in the digestion of protein. For those who have rheumatism a mixture of cucumber juice and carrot juice may be helpful for alleviating the condition. Cucumber juice also has many other uses including possible relief from migraine headaches. When you are feeling tired and need a pick-me-up, eating cucumber with its B vitamins and carbohydrate content will keep you going for hours. Snacking on cucumbers is a healthy way to control the urge for afternoon or evening binge eating.

Aside from its nutritional benefits a slice of cucumber pressed against the roof of your mouth for 30 seconds will eliminate bad breath. It can be used to keep a bathroom mirror from fogging, polish your shoes to a nice shine, stop a squeaky hinge from squeaking, or to polish the tarnish from a stainless steel faucet and sink.

Cucumber has also been found to have cosmetic benefits. It is used in hand and body lotions; mashed cucumber can be applied to the face as a pack to produce a glowing complexion, and thin slices of cucumber can be placed over the eyes to diminish or erase dark circles.

The home gardener has a large variety of cucumbers to choose from. Some are burpless, and some have only small seeds. Others are used for pickling. Cucumber is good in salads, or it can be sliced into a dish with water, a little vinegar, a dash of salt, and a sweetener. A fresh cucumber picked from the garden and eaten like an apple is a refreshing snack.

Sweet Potatoes:

These potatoes are a super food that is starting to be appreciated. Indeed they are worthy of a prominent place in the diet due to the magnitude of their nutritional values and health benefits. There are hundreds of varieties of these tubers misnamed "potatoes", including an orange fleshed variety called "yams". They are much more nutritious than any of the other varieties of potatoes. With 35 grams of complex carbohydrates per serving, sweet potatoes provide more and longer-lasting energy than white potatoes.

Nutritionally, one average sweet potato has 7864.16 mcg of

beta-carotene, a cancer fighting antioxidant that gives them their orange color. Among other benefits this nutrient is helpful in the cognitive function of older men, seemingly aiding verbal memory. They also have a large amount of vitamin A that benefits the immune system along with 306.05 mg of potassium, 17.06 mg of vitamin C, and good amounts of manganese, copper, and vitamin B6. The average adult should consume 4,700 mg of potassium daily. Potassium helps to regulate blood pressure.

Sweet potatoes have at least 4 grams of fiber, which digests slowly causing the stomach to feel full longer. This fiber also helps to lower LDL (bad) cholesterol. A study published in the Archives of Internal Medicine indicates that those who ate the most fiber were 22% less likely to die from any cause compared to those who ate a low fiber diet.

As they provide low insulin resistance they are beneficial to those with diabetes. It is suspected that the low rate of kidney cancer in Asian cultures may be due to their frequent consumption of sweet potatoes.

The best way to enjoy sweet potatoes is baked with the skins on, then cut in half and eat with Smart Balance and honey to taste. Bake only until tender.

Don't store uncooked sweet potatoes in the refrigerator because that is too moist. Instead, store them in a cool, dark place with plenty of ventilation.

Pomegranate:

Here is a fruit with such a host of benefits that nobody could doubt that it is a super food. Pomegranate juice is packed with powerful antioxidants that guard the body in many ways.

Scientists have found that pomegranate contains compounds that have powerful antioxidant and anti-inflammatory abilities that make them protect the cardiovascular system. In tests of a variety of juices, pomegranate was found to be the most effective at inhibiting the damaging effects of free radicals and promoting healthy amounts of nitric oxide. It appears to be effective in keeping a good flow of blood through the carotid arteries in the neck, providing a good flow of blood to the brain thus diminishing the risk of a stroke. This action is so strong that atherosclerosis may actually be reversed and reduce blood pressure.

These benefits may be had by drinking as little as 2 ounces of this juice daily for at least three months.

The benefits of pomegranate do not stop there as it is also beneficial to diabetics and pre-diabetics because it lowers the blood-sugar ratio, preventing the surge sometimes found after meals. Men with prostate cancer should eat pomegranates because they prevent the growth and even lead to the death of the cancerous cells without harming healthy cells; something that chemotherapy does not do. Other benefits include the possible prevention of osteoarthritis and of dental plaque on teeth. This latter benefit may be had by swishing the juice around in the mouth before swallowing..

Extracts of pomegranate appear to protect the skin from ultraviolet light in ways not previously found in other preparations. Check skin creams for this ingredient. Recent discoveries indicate that the antioxidants in pomegranate may protect the liver from stress. It is easy to conclude that the exceedingly powerful antioxidants in pomegranate make it an undisputed super food. Anyone affected by any of these problems would do well to add a little pomegranate to their diet.[26]

Onions:

These aromatic bulbs provide many health benefits including a lot of power for your immune system. They are high in many nutrients beginning with chromium, vitamin C, and dietary fiber, all of which are rated "very good" by nutritional authorities placing them among the world's healthiest foods. They also contain manganese, molybdenum, vitamin B6, tryptophan, folate, potassium, phosphorous and copper, all of which are rated as "good".

Both onions and its relative garlic are members of the Allium family. Allium is a sulfur compound, which gives them their pungent odors. Onions are an outstanding source of the flavonoid polyphenol quercetin, They rank in the top ten among common vegetables with this ingredient. Some onions may provide as much as 100 milligrams of this ingredient. Getting quercetin from this natural source can provide better protection than getting it in a supplement form. Quercitin is an antioxidant that protects our bodies from free radicals. It is known to trigger the ability of the body to produce energy. When onions are cooked over low heat, as in soups, the quercitin is not downgraded but it is transferred into the water.

The amount of polyphenols in onions is higher than in garlic and leeks. In fact, few vegetables have more. Several servings of onions each week will protect a person from the risk of colon and ovarian cancer. One onion serving (½ cup) daily will give maximum protection against these and also oral and esophageal cancers.

When eaten daily with other fruits and vegetables, onion works in synergy to protect the heart and blood vessels. It may also have an anti-clotting capacity in the blood. It is a benefit to menopausal and post-menopausal women in protecting them from loss of bone density. The sulfur content may provide benefits to the body's connective tissue.

Onion has demonstrated anti-inflammatory benefits. It does this by supporting the immune system. This is where the benefits of quercetin are realized. Onions have also been proven to have anti-bacterial benefits when eaten raw. These benefits have been realized in several ways including periodontal disease. It has been noted that those who eat raw onion daily throughout the winter months have little difficulty with colds and flu. . These effects may be because of the powerful *"life force"* in onions. An onion peeled, partially sliced, put in a plastic bag and refrigerated will continue to grow from its core. This demonstrates the *"life force"* that is obtained from eating fresh raw onion. The sulfur compound allicin, an amino acid, may be responsible for this superbiological activity. Onions should be a regular part of every diet.

It is to be noted that a major portion of the beneficial nutrients of onions are in the outer layers just under the skin. When peeling an onion, do not remove any more of the outer portion than necessary.

Asparagus:

Besides its delicious taste Asparagus confers nine distinct health benefits, so it is a worthy health food.

1. It can detoxify the system. Asparagus has often been referred to as a spring tonic because it comes up early in the spring and is so delicious. It has 288 mg of potassium per cup. Potassium is

known for reducing belly fat. (Many of the super foods suggested here are high in potassium). Asparagus also contains 3 g of fiber which cleanses the digestive system. It has no fat or cholesterol. One cup has only 40 calories. It is the ultimate detox vegetable.

2. It has anti-aging functions. Asparagus is high in glutathione, which is an amino acid with potent antioxidant properties, making it a must as an anti-aging deterrent protecting the body's cells.

3. Asparagus is considered an aphrodisiac because of its shape. It is said to trigger the mind to have a physiological response. French grooms in the 19th century were fed three plates of asparagus before their wedding. The large amount of folic acid was thought to increase the production of histamine, necessary for successful love-making. In reality, a good sexual life is healthy in many respects.

4. It functions as a cancer protective because it is high in folate which is known for this important role. Folate is the natural form of folic acid.

5. Reducing pain and inflammation is another benefit of the folate.

6. The folate content also reduces the risk of heart disease.

7. Preventing osteoporosis and osteoarthritis is a benefit of its vitamin K content. Vitamin K is essential for bone formation and repair.

8. It prevents birth defects. While this, admittedly, is not a concern for senior readers, unless you are a Hunzan who can birth children at 80 years of age, it may be a benefit to pass along to your children and grandchildren.

9. Asparagus is known to protect the urinary system from infections (UTI).

Asparagus should be eaten raw to preserve all of the enzymes and nutrients.

Almonds:

Almonds are one of the most nutritious nuts. They have 6g of total carbohydrates and 3 grams of fiber per one ounce serving. A one-ounce serving gives you vitamin E (7.3 mg), folate (8.2 mg), calcium (70 mg), magnesium 78 mg), phosphorus 134 mg), and potassium (206 mg).

Although the serving size contains 163 calories, there are circumstances that make this acceptable for several reasons.

The first of these is the large amount of nutrition packed into almonds. Instead of causing weight gain, they actually promote losing weight, largely due to the high amount of fiber which satisfies the appetite and promotes a long-lasting sense of fullness. Compounds in almonds tend to reduce levels of LDL cholesterol. Almond butter actually not only reduces LDL but also increases HDL, and, because it is lower in saturated fat, it is recommended above peanut butter. Because of their effect on HDL – LDL levels they reduce the risk of cardiovascular disease.

It is most interesting that phytochemicals in nuts are thought to prevent some cancers. Eating nuts reduces the risk of gallstones in men and postmenopausal women. Eating almonds regulates blood glucose levels following meals.

So, when you desire a snack you can munch a handful of almonds without feeling guilty. [27]

Horseradish:

You may be surprised to see horseradish included as a super food, but it is certainly deserving of the honor because it is much more than just a condiment. One thing that can be said about it is that it has known antibiotic properties. It also has good amounts of cancer fighting compounds called *glucosinolates* which make it possible for the liver to detoxify carcinogens and hinder the growth of tumors. While broccoli is known to be a powerful cancer fighter, horseradish may have ten times more glucosinolates than broccoli. Therefore, it appears to be a more potent cancer fighter. Vegetables containing this ingredient are thought to be effective against rectal and colon cancers.

Perhaps also surprising is that horseradish is an effective treatment for sinusitis. A half-teaspoon of the sauce is all it takes. It is important not to drink anything within ten minutes before or after ingesting the sauce.

Horseradish is also effective in treating urinary tract infections (UTI), and it has been found to relieve water retention in the body. With these things in mind, you should no longer be tempted to look down on horseradish since it stands proud of its healthy capabilities.

Grape Juice (purple, unsweetened):

Dr. Martha Grogan, a cardiologist at the Mayo Clinic, reports that purple grape juice made from concord grapes may possibly contain many of the same health benefits as red wine. This juice may reduce the risk of heart disease by relaxing the blood vessels allowing blood to flow more freely. This is due to antioxidants found in the skins of the grapes. Recent studies suggest the following benefits:

1. Reducing the risk of blood clots.
2. Reducing LDL (bad) cholesterol.
3. Preventing damage to blood vessels in the heart.
4. Helping to maintain healthy blood pressure.

Both red wine and the grape juice contain flavonoids and antioxidants which have been shown to increase HDL cholesterol, lowering your risk of atherosclerosis (clogged arteries). It may also help to lower blood pressure.

Some people think that the anti-aging nutrient, resveratrol, only occurs in red wine. This is misunderstanding. Welch's Grape Juice Company confirms that resveratrol is present in their grape juice. Resveratrol is produced in the skin of dark red and purple grapes to protect them from disease. If it is in the skin of the grape then, of course, it is also in grape juice. Fermentation does not create resveratrol, so grape juice contains the polyphenols originally inherent in the grapes. The only difference is that wine is fermented grape juice. The amount of resveratrol may vary by the type of grape. However, commercial grape juice is pasteurized which destroys the enzymes. Freshly made juice has all of the goodness of the grape. Resveratrol is also found in blueberries, cranberries, peanuts and other plants.

To make fresh grape juice, wash the grapes and chop them in a powerful blender (such as a Vita-Mix). Then run the mash through a juicer to fully extract the juice. The result is fresh grape juice made from whole grapes. Fresh juice can be stored in a refrigerator for a few days. If you want to keep the juice longer, it must be processed or frozen to prevent fermentation. Be aware, however, that processing it will destroy the enzymes.

Chapter Eight
Step 2: Exercise

The centenarian George Vrieling had it right when he said that one secret to longevity is to "just keep moving". Our muscles are meant to be used, and that requires movement. One of the great problems of people in America today is that we have become too sedentary. If we don't use our muscles, they tend to atrophy, but when we give them adequate exercise we build strength into them. Exercise is every bit as important for health and longevity as a proper diet is. It is best to exercise daily or at least every other day.

It is generally agreed among exercise authorities that the best form of exercise is simply walking at a reasonable pace that we can sustain for at least 30 minutes. That means not sauntering but just walking at a good steady comfortable pace like you are going someplace and want to arrive in good time. Some folks like to swing their arms while walking, which seems to have some benefit.

In inclement weather, or if for some reason you can't get outside to walk, using a treadmill is a good alternative. Stand upright while you are walking on it and set a good pace that you can maintain for at least 20-30 minutes. You might then get off and do arm or other exercises for a few minutes and then get back on for another 20 minutes.

The second best exercise is bicycle riding. If you have a safe place to ride in a park or on a greenbelt or bike path, you should consider this a good form of exercise for the legs. In fact, bicycling is excellent for strengthening your legs for a backpack trip because it strengthens the knees, which is important for improving your uphill walking and climbing. Vary your speed from fast to faster and then slower again. Nice scenery, possibly with a companion, makes this pleasant exercise. Plan to ride at least 2-3 miles about three times each week. When you are in shape you may enjoy a half-day or longer trip. Take along water and fruit or a granola bar. It would be ideal to walk some days and ride on other days.

A stationary bike is the second-best means of getting this form of exercise. It is more interesting if you can position your bike so that you can look out a window while riding. Of course, if you are in a gym, you can enjoy being with or watching other people. If your bike has a timer and a speedometer-odometer, set the timer for ten minutes and plan to ride two miles in that time with light tension on the wheel. Begin riding at about 12 miles per hour for four minutes, then speed-up to about 15 mph for three minutes, and then drop back to 12 mph for the remainder of your miles. You may want to get off and do another exercise and then get back on and ride another couple miles.

Arm exercises can be done with dumbbells, three pounds for ladies and five pounds for men. The goal is not the weight but the mobility of the exercise. Start by standing erect with the dumbbells at your side, then lift them up to your armpits and back down ten times. Then extend your arms straight out to the sides from your shoulders and bend your elbows up to bring them to your shoulders. Do this ten times. Next extend your arms straight out in front of you and pull the dumbbells back to your chest for ten repetitions. Finally, raise the weights over your head and down to your shoulders for a final ten repetitions. Another exercise you may do with the dumbbells is to stand erect with them by your side and then bend at the hips, down and up for ten repetitions. These are good exercises to do in between your sets of riding the stationary bike.

You do not need to purchase a lot of expensive equipment to get adequate exercise. For example, if you can't get outdoors to walk, you can exercise by standing in-place and raising your feet up and down as if you were walking. Instead of using a stair-stepper, walk up and down a flight of stairs. The next exercises can be done lying down, and we will also explain some exercises to do while sitting.

Lying flat on your back on a firm bed, an exercise table, or a mat, first bend your right leg back to where you can fold your hands around the knee and pull the leg straight back as far as possible, count to three, and then return to the starting position. Then do the same with the left leg and continue for five repetitions with each.

The next exercise rotates your body at the hips. Continuing to lay flat on your back, pull your feet straight back to your buttocks as far as possible. From this position, swing your legs over to the right as far as possible, and hold them there momentarily, then raise them back to the starting position and then over to the left and back up. As you do this count 1-2-3-1, 1-2-3-2, and so on, continuing until you have repeated 10 times. Extend your legs back down for a brief rest.

The next two exercises are good for replacing belly fat with muscle. First, pull your feet up to your buttocks as you did in the previous exercise. This time, with your hands folded across your mid-section, as you exhale contract your lower abdominal muscles as tightly as possible, hold momentarily, then inhale as you relax. This will feel like you are pulling your hips toward your center, but actually you are just contracting your muscles. Your goal will be to continue this for 20 repetitions. Relax and rest a few seconds.

Next, continuing in the same position, while exhaling, raise your head (somewhat like you are trying to do a sit-up) until your shoulders are off the surface and your upper abdominal muscles are contracted as much as possible. Then inhale and relax. Your goal will be to repeat this 10 times. It will seem difficult at first, but it will get easier. As you progress and gain strength, you may be able to repeat this process for another set.

Sitting on the side of the bed or on a solid chair (like a kitchen chair) with your knees slightly spread, while exhaling, bend forward as far as possible to position your head between your knees, hold for a count of five, then inhale and sit up straight. Repeat this five times.

To strengthen your biceps and your neck muscles, do this one. Sitting up straight, interlock the fingers of your hands behind your head. Then simultaneously pull forward with your hands and push your head back to resist with full effort; count to five and relax. Repeat this five times.

Many senior adults tend to develop slumping shoulders and a curvature in the neck. This exercise helps to straighten a curvature of the neck and relax nerve tension. Fold a bath towel in half length-wise; then, roll it up as tightly as possible. Laying flat on your back and with your knees raised, position the towel under your neck so that your head hangs over it and slightly off the surface beneath. Relax and remain in this position for ten minutes.

Another exercise to help eliminate a spinal curvature in the neck is to lay across a bed with your knees up and your head hanging down over the edge. Maintain this position for 5-10 minutes.

While standing straight, bend forward like you are attempting to touch your toes. When you are down as far as possible, without bending your knees, raise up slightly and then down (like you are attempting to touch your toes) up and down five times. You should find that each time you can go down a little farther. Repeat this another time or two. You may find that as you stretch your leg muscles you will actually get to where you can touch your toes. How long has it been since you could do that?

If you are having a problem with sciatica or your lower back, try this. Lying flat on your back but keeping your right leg straight, swing it up as far as possible to a vertical position and then lower it back down. Repeat this five times. But on the fifth time instead of lowering it as before, while keeping your shoulders flat on the laying surface, swing your right leg as far left and down as possible; holding it there, kick five times as if to try to make your foot go farther. Then raise it back to the vertical position and straight down. Repeat this with the left leg swinging it to the right and kicking as before.

Getting lots of fresh air, and some exposure to the sun is essential to health. So, whenever possible, getting your exercise outdoors, by walking, bicycle riding, or participating in some sport, provides a double benefit.

"Bodily exercise profits a little, but godliness is profitable for all things."
1 Timothy 4:8

Chapter Nine
Step 3: Spirituality

The steps of The Longevity Diet plan are not given here in the order of importance. If they were this step should be No. 1 because spirituality fully involves the deepest part – the heart and soul – of man. It is the essential essence of our being. In all of the cultures of the world it has been found that spirituality is central. Every culture recognizes a divine Supreme Being or God, to whom they worship and seek to be obedient. It has been found that this attribute plays a prominent role in the longevity of the longest-lived people. The biographies given earlier in this work attest to this fact.

When Moses delivered the Ten Commandments longevity was in them. They require worship of the one true God and honor to our parents "that your days may be long upon the land" (Ex.20:12). Thus longevity is promised to those of the Judeo-Christian faith.

In the wisdom literature, Solomon teaches, "My child, never forget the things I have taught you. Store my commands in your heart, for "they will give you a long and satisfying life" (Proverbs 3: 1-2 NLT). In another place, he emphasizes, "Wisdom is a tree of life to those who embrace her; happy are those who hold her tightly" (Proverbs 3:18 NLT).

Solomon learned wisdom from his father David, who learned, sometimes the hard way, to live in reverence fully trusting God. In the selections from David's Psalms, quoted here from the New Living Translation, we find the beliefs by which he lived.

Jim Heckathorn

The Creed of David's Life

"The Lord is my Shepherd; I have everything I need. . . He guides me along right paths, bringing honor to His name. . . Even when I walk through the dark valley of death, I will not be afraid, for you are close beside me. Your rod and staff protect and comfort me" (23: 1, 3, 4 NLT).

"Who may climb the mountain of the Lord? Who may stand in His holy Place? Only those whose hands and hearts are pure". . . (24: 3-4).

"To You, O Lord, I lift up my soul. I trust in you my God! . . . Show me the path where I should walk, O Lord; point out the right road for me to follow. Lead me by your truth and teach me, for you are the God who saves me. All day long I put my hope in you. The Lord is good and does what is right; He shows the proper path to those who go astray. He leads the humble in what is right, teaching them His way. The Lord leads with unfailing love and faithfulness all those who keep His covenant and obey His decrees" (25: 1, 4-5, 8-10) NLT.

"I am constantly aware of your unfailing love. . . I have taken a stand, and I will publicly praise the Lord" (26:2, 12 NLT).

"The Lord is my light and my salvation – so why should I be afraid? The Lord protects me from danger – so why should I tremble?" (27:1 NLT).

"The Lord is my strength and my shield from every danger. I trust Him with all my heart. He helps me, and my heart is filled with joy. . . Give honor to the Lord for the glory of His name. Worship the Lord in the splendor of His holiness" (28:7; 29:2 NLT).

"O Lord, I have come to you for protection . . . You are my rock and my fortress. I am overcome with joy because of your unfailing love . . . Love the Lord, all you faithful ones! For the Lord protects those who are loyal to Him" (31: 1a,3a,7a, 23 NLT).

"When I refused to confess my sin, I was weak and miserable, and I groaned all day long. Day and night your hand of discipline was heavy on me. My strength evaporated like water in the summer heat. . . The Lord says I will guide you along the best pathway for your life. I will advise you and watch over you. . . So rejoice in the Lord and be glad, all you who obey Him! Shout for joy, all you whose hearts are pure!" (33:1, 4, 8, 11 NLT).

"The word of the Lord holds true, and everything He does is worthy

174

of our trust. He loves whatever is just and good, and His unfailing love fills the earth" (33:4, 5 NLT).

"Taste and see that the Lord is good. Oh, the joys of those who trust Him! Let the Lord's people show him reverence, for those who honor Him will have all they need . . . those who trust in the Lord will never lack any good thing. . . *Do any of you want to live a life that is long and good?* Turn away from evil and do good. Work hard at being at peace with others. . . The righteous face many troubles, but the Lord rescues them from each and every one" (34: 8-10, 12, 14, 19 NLT, emphasis added).

These verses, in a nutshell, reveal the spiritual ideals that motivated David's life. He attributed all to the love of God and to trusting Him for everything. It is the same way with the long-lived seniors that have been interviewed for this work. They have lived faithful lives, and the Lord has rewarded them with His joy and length of days.

The Spiritual Effect:

Longevity requires a holistic view of human nature. As the spiritual aspect is the most real part of man, the soul that is at peace with God will rest joyfully in the satisfaction of that relationship with God.

Studies have shown people find spiritual satisfaction in various faiths. However, spirituality is most explicitly and satisfactorily developed in Christianity. David stated the benefits as forgiveness, healing of diseases, redemption, lovingkindness, tender mercies and the satisfaction of good things, so that your youth is renewed like the eagle's," (Psalm 103: 2-5). When non-believers or adherents of other faiths learn what Christianity truly offers them, they frequently leave their old way of believing to embrace Christianity. Along with the benefits David set forth it is the love of Christ that woos them. In Him is found the hope that overcomes all hopelessness.

The ultimate truth found to be at the core of Christianity is the love of God. When asked what he considered to be ultimately the most important commandment, Jesus responded, "You shall love the Lord your God with all your heart, with all your soul, and with all your mind. . . And the second is like it: 'You shall love your neighbor as yourself" (Matt. 22-37-40). When asked how people could know "the way", Jesus, the Christ, said, "I am the way the truth and the life. No one comes to the Father except through me" (John 14:6). "I have come that they may have life and that they may have it more abundantly" (John 10:10). In Christianity, men and women find abundance of truth and true longevity both in quantity and quality of years. Through Jesus, the love of God is revealed as a divine, intimate, loving relationship.

It remains for each individual to attain the wisdom to discern, desire, and appropriate into his life the fullness of this love that is freely offered. People who have the love of God in their hearts will have love for other people, and that love desires the very best for everyone, (1 John 4:7-11). As David said, "Work hard at being at peace with others". It's the love of God in our hearts that makes this possible. It was this love that made David the most loved and successful of the kings of Israel.

A love relationship with God cannot be effectively maintained on a casual basis. That is, one cannot merely assent to accepting and loving Christ as a personal Savior and proceed in a daily walk that is not fully committed to seeking His way of life. John wrote, "If we say that we have fellowship with Him, and walk in darkness, we lie and do not practice the truth. But if we walk in the light as He is in the light, we have fellowship with one another," (1 John 1:6-7). A love relationship with the Lord is akin to a spousal relationship. If a husband does his best to considerately maintain an intimate loving relationship, caring for the needs of his wife, his wife will respond likewise to care for the needs of the one who is so loving to her. If a person intimately loves the Lord, the Lord will provide for the one who demonstrates true love.

Prayer is provided, first and foremost, as a means of conversing and building an intimate relationship with our Heavenly Father. Yet, too often we look upon it as a means of begging for blessings that the Father already knows about and will freely give to those who intimately demonstrate love to Him. Reading about God's ways and words to man in the Bible is provided to facilitate an intimate relationship with the Godhead. Reading the psalms of David reveals how he established an intimate relationship with God.

There is much more to the love of God than humans can understand if we look at it only on the human level. Humans must rise to the divine to understand "the width and length and depth and height – to know the love of Christ that passes (human) knowledge" and fills the heart with the fullness of God (Eph. 3:18-19). This is what we see in the creed of David's life. The love of God lifted him to full devotement to God, and his right relationship with God which provided his deep inward joy.

Long years before David, Moses had enjoined the Israelites to love God as the basic tenet of faith, but they did not fully understand and embrace this truth. It remained for Jesus to emphasize the commands to love God and our neighbor as ourselves, and to demonstrate this love by the life He lived. As He said, "Greater love has no one than to lay down one's life for His friends" (John 15: 13), which is exactly what He did for mankind. By His sacrifice as the "Lamb of God" He purchased our salvation and opened the doors of heaven for us. What more could anyone desire than that which is offered through the love of God? The gratification of selfish desires cannot equal what God's love offers. Those who make this discovery will know the way to live long and live well.

When a person is fully engrossed in a lifestyle of love he finds true meaningfulness and purpose in living. Far greater than this is the promise of continued longevity, eternally, through the life of the Spirit. Jesus said, "I am the resurrection and the life. He who believes in Me, though he may die, he shall live, and. *never die,*" (John 11:25, 26, emphasis added). A person who values life will value the promise of eternal life.

Living a loving lifestyle is the pathway to eternal life. One must learn to look consistently upon the situations of life by asking himself or herself, "What is the most loving manner in which I can respond to this situation?" In this manner the Holy Spirit will lead a person to appropriate the love of God as his or her own loving nature. Life will be worth living and the transition to a heavenly home will be the fruition of joy that has been established in this life. First comes the beauty of the blossom and then the sweetness of the fruit, but these come only through cultivation. Live in such a way that you are nurturing your soul for eternity.

> *"To love is to take on the likeness of God for, "God is Love".*
> *Therefore, everything we want God to be to us, by His grace,*
> *we must also be to others."*   Jim Heckathorn

> *"Life is a journey into love, it seems to me, and there's nothing so*
> *beautiful as a godly soul. Physical exercise is good, no doubt, but*
> *there is something far, far better: It is to love."*[28]   David Roper

Chapter Ten
Step 4: Stress Management and Rest

These are being combined because they work together to rejuvenate the body. An important asset in stress management is to get adequate rest and recreation. The importance of eight hours of sleep nightly cannot be overemphasized. Those who get by on six hours of sleep have formed a habit in which they simply "get by". They find that eventually, they need to find a day to sleep-in. It has been said that each hour of sleep before midnight is worth two hours after midnight. The hours late in the day are not usually the best time to be productive. Those who arise early find that they can productively face a new day with a clear mind and rested body. The old adage is very appropriate, "Early to bed and early to rise makes a man healthy, wealthy and wise.

Those who can, especially senior citizens, will find it helpful to take naps and practice a low stress lifestyle such as we found to be the practice of the Mediterranean people of Ikaria. Another good practice of these people is to be laid-back about things as they go through the day. So to say, "take time to smell the flowers." Stop to visit with a friend or to give help to someone in need. Recreational activities with family or friends, just for fun, on a regular basis, re-creates both body and soul. These may include sports, fishing, hiking, golf, or another outdoor activity. Outdoor activities are best because they take you away from the ordinary habits and routines of life to get fresh air and sunshine which are also necessary to good health. An individual can face life better when the mind and body are in healthy condition.

Stress can be the most debilitating aging factor that a person must deal with. It encroaches upon the life of every individual to "upset the apple cart" of a peaceful existence. Often a person may not consciously be aware of stress but none can avoid it. Stress comes when we are frustrated in actualizing the needs, desires and goals of our lives. A person may be doing his very best to actualize his life harmoniously but will still come upon situations that cause stress.

Some of the things that cause stress are personal things; financial difficulty, choices to be made with ambivalent options, mechanical problems with your vehicle at what seems to be the worst possible time, the difficulties that must be endured to obtain some goal, perhaps a legal matter, problems caused by sickness and disease that may be life threatening, the death of a loved one, or worse still relational problems with close family or friends, or a marriage ending in divorce. Many of these things cut to the core of our being.

Many things that cause extreme stress are caused by natural disasters such as storms, floods, or fire. Others may be circumstances causing financial hardship caused by a downturn in the economy, the loss of employment, or stresses caused by war may cause some, too. Some in our study were prisoners of war.

Other stresses may come upon us due to guilt and loss of self-esteem for our personal behavior, the violation of spiritual, social, or moral values or of some law. Bad habits can cause stress even if they just lead to our neglecting to get enough sleep or being a workaholic.

The effect of stress upon a person's life will depend upon the duration of the stressful situation and his or her attitude or the manner in which the individual looks upon, accepts and manages the stressful situation. Christians turn to their faith to get them through stressful times. In every circumstance of life it bolsters a person emotionally and spiritually to always do your best and be your best. Seeking honorable ways to manage your stresses will create within you emotional and spiritual strength to endure the stresses you encounter.

In his book, "Making Stress Work for You", Lloyd J. Ogilvie points out the importance of a daily time of prayerful meditation as a means of overcoming the stresses of life:

"At a crucial time in Jesus' ministry when He and His disciples were being besieged by the needs of people, He said, "Come aside by yourselves to a deserted place and rest awhile" (Mark 6:30). The words actually mean, "Come away for yourselves and rest awhile." The Lord wants us to love ourselves as loved by Him and give ourselves the gift of time each day for stress-reducing communion with Him. An unwillingness to meditate each day may be an expression of self-affirmation. Why else would we deny ourselves the time to lower our stress level and become prepared to live more abundantly?"

Ogilvie continues,

"The important thing that a daily time of meditation makes possible is the actual change of our mental attitudes as well as our bodily response. We place ourselves at the disposal of the healing Spirit of the Lord. James asks, "Is anyone suffering? Let him pray. Is anyone cheerful? Let him sing psalms" (James 5:13). Actually, creative meditation includes both prayer for our suffering and praise for the Lord's help in spite of everything. We can talk to Him about the difficulties and delights of life. He helps us overcome our hard times of suffering and truly enjoy our times of praise. And soon the praise over His interventions gives us a hopeful resiliency for the future."[29]

Jake DeShazer, who was one of the Doolittle Raiders that bombed Japan early in World War II, was captured when his plane went down, and he was held as a prisoner of the Japanese for three and one-half years. His treatment was often not good; many died while imprisoned. Jake survived his imprisonment by dependence upon God. As he meditated and prayed while in the prison, he even found love in his heart for the Japanese people which caused him to return to Japan as a Christian missionary. Being a prisoner of war changed the course of his life. He devoted his life to living and serving in the love of God. Although he suffered the hardship of being a prisoner of war and experienced many frustrations, his dependence upon God kept him going until March 15, 2008, when he died at 96 years of age. Frank Buckles, who was also a prisoner of the Japanese throughout the war, died in February 2011, having lived to be 110 years old.

Stress has a holistic effect upon the whole body. If a person lives in worry and fear; harbors bad attitudes, such as anger, grief, and resentment, stress will take a terrible toll upon the person's life causing that person's aging process to accelerate. Looking upon one's difficulty with a wise perspective which sees a good aspect to a situation tends to give some sense of peace in the midst of the turmoil. A person's state of mind will determine the damage to the body and its lifespan. Stress should summon a person to use his or her inner resources to overcome the stressful situation by doing and being one's very best self. It has been found that those who accept their stress with wholesome attitudes and find wholesome ways to manage their stress are less adversely affected by the stresses of life. These are people who depend upon their deep faith in God for strength, courage and guidance both to endure and to look for a bright outcome. When stress is caused by another person, one must look within to find love and forgiveness. This is the course that is uplifting. One cannot allow the acts of others to be a drag upon one's life. A person can actually manage the stresses of life creatively and wholesomely to emerge victoriously as a better person.

Finally, be aware that stress can be caused by the use of tobacco products, alcohol consumption, and a diet including eating excess fatty foods and sweets. Although these stresses are physical rather than emotional, all forms of stress take a toll on the body and should be prevented as much as possible. I have noted that those who live the longest have been careful to avoid these stress factors.

Supplements that have been found to offer "powerful protection against stress and anxiety through distinct and complementary mechanisms, are lemon balm and L-theanine. Both have been shown to reduce not only stress but the biological manifestations it produces in the body and brain."[30] Vitamin C has also long been held to be helpful in relieving stress.

It has been observed that a husband and wife that live a harmonious, happy life can very possibly live long lives. There are two reasons for this. First, is that they manage the stress in their lives very well. The other reason is that they have the comfort of snuggling together when they go to bed. Snuggling is a great stress reliever, and is conducive to the most restful deep sleep. Human Growth Hormone (hGH), which is the master hormone of youthfulness, is released from the pituitary gland while they are lovingly getting peaceful deep sleep. Regretfully, those whose senior years are lonely don't have this benefit.

As it affects a huge proportion of our population in some manner, stress is a very serious aging factor making it essential for adults to use all the means at their disposal to recognize and cope with it.

Chapter Eleven
Step 5: Family and Social Life

It has been noted that one important aspect that helps to maintain a happy wholesome lifespan is the relationships that an aging person has with immediate family, extended family, and with friends. One of the greatest needs of aging adults is to associate regularly with people to whom they can relate, in whose company they can have pleasant and enjoyable experiences, and with whom they can laugh or cry. There needs to be, at least, one person with whom an individual can have pleasant conversation and experiences on a regular basis. There is a saying, "We don't stop laughing because we grow old, we grow old because we stop laughing."

There are some essential factors involved in building wholesome lasting relationships with family and friends. The first is to develop love in your life so that you will love other people. Love begets love, so love extended to others is well invested. When you love others, you desire the best for them. You reach out to them with the thoughtfulness of a caring heart to do kind deeds or labors of love when you see another with a need. You compliment others and rejoice with them in their successes; and you grieve with them over losses or failures. Love seeks to be interested and understanding of the circumstances in the lives of family members and friends. It is always kind, considerate, and willing to forgive if offended. We can share good times with those we love. If you desire loving relationships you must cultivate a loving heart that reaches out to others.

Honor and respect are also essential for cultivating wholesome relationships. Everybody appreciates a friend or family member who demonstrates honor and respect. It is important to you and your friends to know that you are held in high regard and that your friendship is important and valued. These things lift a relationship to its highest level.

Another quality of solid relationships is loyalty. This is the quality that binds a relationship. We all need those who will stand by us to help and encourage us and who will be there for us when we need them most. To have such friends, we must show ourselves to be such a friend.

The Scrivners are a good example of a happily married couple who lived in their own home and enjoyed the love and companionship that each provided for the other until he was past 100 years of age. When Bev Shea's wife died, he lived for ten years without a spouse, but he had the close association of those with whom he worked in ministry. In 1985, he was delighted to again have a wife to share his life, and they were together in their own home for over 26 years. He continued to do well at 102 years of age with the help of his delightful spouse.

When a man loses his wife, it is usually important for him to find another spouse. Man was created with the innate need for a female companion; therefore, he finds a lonely existence to be stressful such that it will shorten his lifespan. Women seem to have the ability to manage a bit better by finding fellowship with family and close friends or even with a pet.

Perceived loneliness is one of the most debilitating factors of aging. Lonely people have higher levels of cortisol and inflammation. Loneliness has also been shown to make it harder for blood to move through the arteries, which raises blood pressure.[31] Some individuals seem to manage quite well alone, while others require a lot of close companionship. Having a connection at appropriate times is very important.

Senior adults look forward to fellowship times with family at holidays and for special events. Especially if one has lost a spouse, these times of family fellowship are anticipated to lift the spirit by knowing that someone cares for them. We have found that the Japanese have a social system which highly values, honors, and respects aging parents and grandparents; younger family members frequently gather with them on weekends and special occasions to have joyful times. With this traditional value system, aging seniors find considerable pleasure that blesses their years. In America, a similar closeness exists with some families, and it would be well for more to adopt this social pattern for the well-being and benefits to both old and young.

Often, uplifting associations are provided through the church or an organization to which the person is a member and to which the individual has a sense of belonging. This situation works best when the aging senior is still mobile and can drive a vehicle or have transportation provided.

One of the saddest events in the life of a senior is when one must live alone without frequent contact with family or when a senior has little, or no, choice other than to live in a retirement home. Here the individual is separated from familiar friends and all too often is seldom or infrequently visited by family members. This is a very stressful situation for the one who must endure such circumstances, and the individual often sinks into a state of depression. This situation causes some to regress emotionally and physically. When George Vreiling moved away from the farm into a retirement home with his wife because she needed some help, he lived only about four months in this new environment. He had not been sick; he just laid back and went to be with the Lord.

In earlier times, when children took their aging parents into their homes to care for them, this offered a better situation for the seniors, although it sometimes created some problems for the children. There are some who are outgoing and can manage the retirement home scenario better than others. While there are many excellent retirement homes, it is unfortunate that the quality of care in retirement homes varies, with some being sub-standard. It is noted that there are many centenarians, mostly women, living in retirement homes.

Our research indicates that senior adults enjoy the close association of family and friends, especially a spouse. With good fellowship, they are more happily situated to live without the stresses that living alone creates, so they have the opportunity to live longer in a peaceful environment.

Keep Romance Alive: It is so often assumed that in the later years of life our existence will become hum-drum; that romance and the ability to please one's spouse will diminish and perhaps become non-existent. Such thoughts and expectations can cause this to become a self-fulfilling prophecy because some just give-up. This need not occur! The evidence is that most seniors do not lose interest in romance and sexuality as they grow older. Indeed the desire is often intensified.

Due to the loss of a spouse by death or divorce, romance and an active sex life will cease to exist, but studies show that most seniors maintain, at least, a moderate interest in this aspect of life. Although they may think it impossible, some who have experienced a vibrant romantic life maintain high hopes of rediscovering it even as they grow into their 70's, 80's, and 90's. The numbers of seniors who subscribe to online dating clubs attests to this. A truly loving heart seeks to embrace love throughout an individual's lifetime. True love never dies! Romantic desires and physical expressions of love can be satisfactorily achieved by tenderly kissing, hugging, cuddling, caressing, and touching. Thoughtful tenderness is an essential aspect of romance.

The brain is the control center for this, just as it is for all other areas of life. Mental attitude and desire created by deep love is the basic requirement for keeping romance, libido, and sexuality alive in an individual's life. Where a man and a woman have cherishing love for each other, this can continue throughout their lifetimes. Diminishing hormone levels of DHEA and testosterone and increasing bad estrogen levels can be a challenge to an individual's sexuality, but with caring, love can continue as vibrantly in our advanced years as in our youth. Love is the key to keeping romance alive.

Loving thoughtfulness and consideration, smiles, kind words, compliments, tender touches, gentleness, and kindness can continue forever. Candlelight dinners, cards, flowers, gifts, backrubs, or foot rubs, and hugging, holding hands, and cuddling will always be accepted as expressions of tender loving care. It is these expressions of love performed throughout the day and night that express sensuality and keeps love alive.

Due to diminishing testosterone and the testosterone-estrogen balance, many men experience a loss in their manliness. Testosterone replacement therapy using injections, patches or creams has proven successful for many. Although considered off-label for women's hormone problems, some doctors prescribe this successfully for them also. Diidolymethane (DIM), derived from cruciferous vegetables, promotes beneficial estrogen metabolism for both men and women. There are also supplements that some have found to be useful. Doctors can help with other problems. Following the Longevity Diet plan to maintain basic health and vitality is essential for this as in all other areas of our well-being.

While it may be necessary for a couple to adjust to some different ways of touching and pleasing one's spouse, it is still possible for them to fully satisfy each other. With willing desire, they can experiment to find what is most satisfying. It is essential that they have open communication, telling each other what feels good and what doesn't, to find satisfaction while making adjustments in this deeply intimate part of their relationship.

Romantic love is a God-given, essential part of maintaining zestfulness in life, and men and women are rightly driven to fulfill this desire. Whatever the obstacles, don't give up! Where there is a will, there is a way for couples to keep romance alive in their lives.

The legacy of a life.

When a person becomes deceased it is a good thing if he/she can leave a good legacy which allows the deceased to continue to live in the hearts of the individual's family. Some individuals choose to leave a testimonial expressing what life has meant to them and their love and appreciation for those who remain. Some do this in a written testimonial, and others may leave it as a recorded message, while still others leave a video to be viewed and later cherished. A video may include some photos depicting meaningful people, places and events of the person's life and can also include a musical background.

We like the old-fashioned custom of having a visitation night at the home or funeral home where the deceased lies in state. These are good times of fellowship in which family, relatives, and friends can not only pay their respects for the deceased by sharing memories of her or him but also catch-up on current happenings in their lives. A good feature of the funeral service is the opportunity for family members and close friends to express their memories and their appreciation for the character and achievements of the deceased. By these means, the deceased leaves a legacy of love and character to the hearts of loved ones.

Chapter Twelve
Step 6: Maintaining Healthy Youthful Skin

When a person looks into the face of an aging individual, there is an immediate impression of the individual's age and well-being. Individuals that spend much time in outdoor activities all year are constantly exposing their skin to the elements. Without proper skin care, their faces become weathered and deeply wrinkled. It's entirely possible for individuals to appear twenty years older than their actual age. Emotional stress over an extended period will also cause aging that will be reflected in an individual's face and make the individual appear older. For optimal health, it is important to take appropriate care of the skin.

It's possible for individuals who properly care for their skin to appear to be many years younger than their actual age. Healthy skin is an indication of a healthy body. Eating a Mediterranean-style diet such as The Longevity Diet will help to create healthy-looking skin. Research has shown that there are a few nutrients that are especially helpful to the skin. These are: zinc, Omega-3 fatty acids, selenium, vitamin A, vitamin B5, vitamin C, vitamin D, vitamin E, and collagen.

Beauty comes from within in many respects. The body is holistic, so peace and good nutrition within will reflect in the face. While it is possible for a lady using cosmetics to make herself appear lovely, a preferable goal is to maintain a naturally pleasing complexion. A smooth complexion is equally important for men.

In addition to diet, it is important to maintain healthy skin by cleansing and moisturizing the skin. Following is a facial technique suggested by an eye physician that is appropriate for both men and women. First, carefully cleanse the skin using a mild cleanser such as head-to-toe baby wash. Be careful to cleanse around the eyes, nose and ears. Carefully dry the skin without excessive rubbing. Then apply a skin moisturizer, being careful not to get it in the eyes but to cover the areas around the ends of the eyes where crow's feet occur. Also apply moisturizer to the outer portions of the ears. This technique will promote healthy skin and also prevent, or treat, blephartis, which is an itchy irritation of the eyes.

Many men typically use an after-shave lotion. These lotions usually contain some form of alcohol, which is drying to the skin. It is much better to use a skin moisturizer to nourish the skin after shaving.

Skin moisturizers are the single most important thing to apply to the skin to get a healthy, vibrant, youthful appearance. Many people have a favorite product. Hunza women use apricot on their skin, and apricot scrubs are popular with many today. One lady in her seventies who appeared at least ten years younger than her age gave the credit to Pond's Skin Cream. Another lady who maintained a nice complexion preferred Nivea Body Skin Firming Moisturizer. In a conversation this author had with a dermatologist he approved of this product.

The expensive skin treatments and chemical-laden products on the market are not the best way to obtain healthy, youthful looking skin. Our research leads us to prefer a few products containing natural ingredients including collagen, CoQ10, hyaluronic acid, and vitamin E that offer positive results without exceptionally great expense or a long wait to see results.

The Beauty Review 2011 Beauty Awards tested dozens of products by actual use and scored them according to visible results; they reported the results on May 15, 2011. The leading product was "The Solution 5-in-One Skin Complex" by Envision Beauty. This product combines a moisturizer, anti-aging serum, eye cream, and make-up base to make the 5-in-one product. Although this product is a bit costly, the price is not so bad when you consider that it's the only thing you need to purchase to have lovely skin. The judges reported that, "After only a few days using it the skin was noticeably soft and glowing." This product contains 100% natural ingredients and is paraben free. The ingredients are DMAE, alpha lipoic acid, hyaluronic acid, sodium PCA, organic açaí, organic goji, centella asiatica, and vitamins A, B5, C, and E.

Another natural product that scored well was Burt's Bees Body Wash. Still other excellent natural products are Orange Blossom Cleansing Milk and Herbal Nova Crème. Both are formulated for aging and dry skin and are distributed by Scriptures.

One of the greatest concerns regarding skin problems is avoiding skin cancers, so some information addressing this issue is included here. Some of the following is repetitious, but it is worth repeating. Some of these treatments also apply to other forms of cancer.

Skin cancers (actinic keratoses, basal, and squamous) are caused by excess exposure to the sun, and they are highly treatable. Rather ironically, the thing that causes skin cancer also produces one of the things that the body needs most. Exposure to the sun allows the body to produce vitamin D. Recent research has revealed that the human body needs much more vitamin D than medical science had previously thought. Vitamin D is essential for building the immune system and warding off many diseases. It also aids in the absorption of calcium, which is crucial for maintaining bone density. Since our bodies create less vitamin D as we grow older, supplementation is often necessary. Supplementation is also recommended for individuals who live in northern latitudes and for those who have limited exposure to the sun. Doctors who practice natural medicine now recommend that adults take a daily dose of 400 IUs of this important vitamin. Even larger doses, as high as 40,000 IUs, are not harmful when taken over a short period when the body is stressed by illness.

Dark-skinned people require more exposure to the sun to produce vitamin D. Black human skin is thicker than white skin and consequently transmits only about 40% of the UV rays needed for vitamin D to be produced. Many people who have cancers are vitamin D deficient. Black women with skin cancer have been found to be at 7.5 times higher risk of developing other cancers. There is suspicion that black- skinned people may have difficulty producing enough vitamin D to support an immune system strong enough to ward off cancer. Since Vitamin D is essential to healthy skin but black people have a problem producing vitamin D, it seems that a deficiency of vitamin D may contribute to the occurrence of skin cancers. Therefore, vitamin D_3 supplements would be beneficial to black people for the prevention and treatment of all forms of cancer. The irony is that, in black people, the sun damages the skin without producing enough vitamin D to build an immune system strong enough to combat skin cancer.

Diet

A strong immune system is necessary for a healthy body. Choosing a healthy diet is the best way to build a viable immune system, and a vegan diet has been found to be the healthiest. Lorraine Day, MD.[32], who nearly died of breast cancer and cured herself with a vegan diet, has been a strong proponent of the vegan diet to prevent and treat not only cancer but also many other diseases. One important aspect of the vegan diet is to eat most of it as raw vegetables and fruit.

The reason that eating raw vegetables and fruit is so important is that heating food to a temperature above 115 degrees destroys the enzymes, and the enzymes are the life factor in food. Uncooked onions or potatoes will sprout due to the life factor, the enzymes in them. You can slice half of an onion and put the rest in a plastic bag placed in the refrigerator, and the next day you will observe a sprout. The enzymes are actually every bit as important as the vitamins and minerals in your food.

Enzymes should be eaten on an empty stomach so that they can get into the blood stream better. The best benefits are found in cruciferous vegetables (such as broccoli, and cabbage), green leafy vegetables, apples, oranges, black or red grapes, cherries, apricots, plums, and blueberries, but grains and nuts (especially almonds) are also wholesome. Drink fresh fruit and vegetable juices. Carrot juice is a good source of vitamin A, which promotes healing.

Dr. Johanna Budwig discovered a cure for cancer that calls for a twice-daily dose of low-fat cottage cheese (one-half cup) and raw, cold pressed, unrefined linseed oil with lignans (one tablespoon) with perhaps some chopped vegetables added. I like a smoothie made with fruit, low-fat plain yogurt and fresh ground flax seed which may work as well especially as a preventive. It is untested as a treatment as far as I know, but it is delicious and contains lots of enzymes and other nutrients. The secret of Dr. Budwig's plan is that it provides some essential nutrients; however, it is a departure from a strict vegan diet.[33]

Keratoses (pre-cancers) can be easily treated with liquid nitrogen. These appear as scaly spots on the skin. These can advance to become basal or squamous cancers. Dermatologists typically treat keratoses with liquid nitrogen contained in a canister about ten inches tall and three inches in diameter with a special sprayer on top. The sprayer delivers a very brief narrow directional spray to the affected area. The extremely cold nitrogen burns the area sprayed, which then scabs over and eventually drops off. The treatment is quite tolerable for adults but would likely cause small chilren to cry. Glycoalkaloid products have been found to be highly effective on these keratoses, and oil of oregano applied topically has also been found to be effective. Several internet sources offer glycoalkaloid creams. Just search using the word "skin" along with "glycoalkaloids"

Graviola is one of the most effective natural treatments for all forms of cancer. It comes from the Amazon rain forests and is available as capsules for internal use and also a liquid for topical application. Graviola has been highly researched and one lab tried unsuccessfully to reproduce it chemically so they could patent it and make a fortune. It has been found to be 10,000 times stronger than a chemotherapy drug used for breast cancer. Graviola will kill all of the cancer cells without damaging any healthy cells. Several suppliers for this product can be found online. I prefer products available from Rain-Tree Pharmacy, but that may be just a personal preference. Graviola Max may have a broader, more effective spectrum than regular graviola. The topical form is called N-Tense and comes in a two ounce bottle. Graviola is very inexpensive. Full information can be found on the website www.rain-tree.com including research and the various products.[34]

Basal cell and squamous cell are the most common skin cancers and are recognized as small lumps or sore spots that don't heal properly. They are not life-threatening unless they are left untreated for many years. These are typically removed surgically. Chemical compounds known as glycoalkaloids have now been developed that are highly successful. One product called **SkinAnswer** appears to target only the cancerous cells. It is applied twice daily after rubbing with a washcloth to remove dead skin and is usually not covered with a bandage. It works quickly to replace diseased cells with healthy ones. SkinAnswer is a cost-effective product.

This product will remove most any skin problem including moles, skin tags, and liver spots. It is available at some pharmacies and by mail order. It is produced by Compassionet, P.O. Box 710, Saddle River, NJ 07458, phone 1-800-510-2010, Ext. 474.

Vitamin C can also be used successfully to remove basal cell carcinomas. It can be mixed by adding a small amount of water to powdered vitamin C. This paste is applied directly to the spots. After three applications each day for two weeks, most of the spots will scab over and drop off.

Green Tea contains polyphenols that have a strong antioxidant activity that helps to protect DNA against damage. The polyphenols are also effective in blocking the cancer-causing activity of nitrates and nitrites. Drinking green tea before a meal that contains these is recommended. People who drink several cups of green tea daily on a regular basis have a lower occurrence of cancer than other people who drink other teas or no tea.

Green tea is effective in preventing several kinds of cancers including colon, prostate, breast, lung, ovarian, bladder, and skin cancers. Drinking green tea may be a very practical means of cancer prevention. Green tea has several other health benefits including weight loss and detoxification, and the polyphenols it contains also protect heart health because they lower LDL "bad cholesterol" while raising HDL "good cholesterol". Green tea also acts as a natural blood thinner which can lower blood pressure.

Chapter Thirteen
Step 7: Maintaining Mental Attitude and Acuity

One of the most unfortunate things that can happen to a person is losing mental acuity. In losing that, the person loses his personhood. The old-fashioned term for this disability is senility. Today it is called dementia which means "deprived of mind". Dementia affects approximately 6.8 million people in the United States. There are various forms of dementia, but the most common one is Alzheimer's disease (AD). People who have this disease usually live 8-10 years after it is diagnosed, but some live as long as 20 years.

Dementia describes various symptoms including diminished intellectual functioning (memory, movement, language, judgment, behavior and abstract thinking) which interferes with normal life functions. Exhibiting a single symptom such as memory loss does not mean that a person has dementia. There must be at least, two or more symptoms for such a diagnosis. AD can affect relatively young adults as well as elderly people. Dementia is not a normal part of the aging process. Many men and women live well into their nineties and even past 100 years of age without any sign of this problem.

With many types of dementia, nerve cells stop functioning and die. This does not occur with normal aging. AD is caused by amyloid plaques and neurofibrillary tangles in the brain. Scientists are uncertain what causes these to occur. The actual causes of dementia remain a mystery, but genes play a role in some types of dementia. This does not mean that a person is predestined to it, but only that a person may have a predisposition by certain inherited factors. There is so much that is not known that this predisposition is not even clearly defined. Also, there are no drugs that can stop or reverse AD although some may provide temporary relief of some symptoms. Studies have revealed risk factors for dementia, some of which are related to lifestyle. These include smoking, excessive alcohol consumption, atherosclerosis (plaque in arteries), high levels of LDL cholesterol, high levels of homocysteine in the blood, diabetes, and mild cognitive impairment which carries a 40% risk.

Given these risk factors, prevention dictates that individuals who are diabetic or pre-diabetic need to control their glucose levels carefully. Blood testing at regular intervals is required to determine homocysteine and cholesterol levels so that measures can be taken to correct them if they are too high. It's also important to control inflammation in the body.

Diet is essential to control the health of the brain and the body. This brings us again to emphasize the holistic nature of human beings which must be considered to maintain the wholeness of man. Every aspect of body, mind, and soul is interrelated with other aspects, and all must be taken into consideration together to make a healthy being. Diet nourishes the brain as well as the body, and a healthy brain can nourish the soul.

Victor Marchione, M.D., writing for Lombardi "Doctors Health Press", has written a special report in which he indicates some Brain-Boosting Foods. He states, "Your brain pretty much controls everything that happens in your body." He continues, "Fortunately, even though the brain is an amazing complex and sophisticated part of you, it is still just an organ. You can keep your brain healthy, just like your heart or your liver, by eating foods that nourish it. Brain-boosting foods can have a real and lasting impact when it comes to keeping thinking skills sharp and memory intact."[35]

Most of the foods that he includes in his list are discussed in our diet section or as super foods. These include berries, fish, green tea, leafy greens and olive oil.

You may have heard the saying, "If you don't use it, you'll lose it". That is very true concerning our bodies. Athletes must constantly train to maintain their athletic ability. It also applies to the faculties of the brain. If we don't constantly use them, they begin to atrophy. Senior adults have found many ways to keep their bodies and brains functioning well. Being a couch potato is not one of them. Couch potatoes don't grow; they just sit and rot away.

Farmers keep both body and mind active with their varied farming activities. You may not be a farmer, but perhaps you could be a gardener. You could plant vegetables and flowers around your home or, if you don't have much space, you could volunteer to help beautify a city park or to help another who is less capable than you. Being a good neighbor will give you a good sense of satisfaction. George Vreiling and Frank Buckles stayed healthy and alert while working on their farms past the age of 100 years.

Exercise not only is good for the body but also benefits the mind because it helps to stimulate the flow of blood throughout your system. If you can't get outdoors to walk and don't have access to a gym, try going to a shopping mall early or late in the day when it's not crowded to speed walk the open area. Exercise helps to stimulate the production of chemicals called growth factors that aid the neurons of the brain. Go back to the section on exercise for other suggestions.

Education is a good option. Many people are inquisitive by nature and always want to learn something new. If there is a college in your area, you could audit classes for a modest fee. Classes are also available to take on the internet. If you travel internationally or have other nationals in your area you may want to learn another language so that you can converse with them. This always excites them to know that you cared enough to learn their language. It really facilitates relationship. Nola Ochs made it into the Guinness Book of World Records by graduating from Fort Hays State University in Kansas when she was 98 years old. As she approached 100 years of age, she continued to live on campus and pursue her studies for a time, but later went back to enjoying life on the farm with her family.

Reading and writing are two more good ways to keep your mind active. Read about things that interest you, and read to keep informed. There is always a need to write letters to senators and representatives or to send letters to the editor; writing short stories might even be profitable. You could volunteer to read stories to children at the public library or at your local school. Charles Scrivener published his last book when he was 95 years old.

You could get some family members or friends to play games that involve using your mental faculties. Try Scrabble or other word games; chess can be challenging, as can checkers. Alone you can solve crossword puzzles. Choose games that are intellectually stimulating. Perhaps you could find friends at a community center who would like to join you in this activity.

There are always organizations that are looking for volunteers to help with jobs. Contact hospitals, care homes, and your church for ideas. Being involved in your community will not only keep you active but also give you a sense of satisfaction.

If there is a YMCA or exercise club in your area, this is another place you can keep active. If you are still quite agile you could participate in Senior Olympics. These are organized in most states, and there are even national contests.

If you have musical talent such as singing or playing an instrument, this is a good activity to pursue in retirement. A 75 year old lady, Barbera Hartley, recently won first place in a singing contest with a lot of younger competition. Jerry Tlucek, a retired farmer, took up the guitar, started writing and singing songs, then recorded them and traveled to have concerts. Ivis Meitler, a pianist, became a recording artist at 100 years of age. Bev Shea, at 102 years of age, still played his piano and organ and went through the day with a song in his heart. If you have talent pursue your possibilities.

Music is relaxing and uplifting to the soul. If you go through your day with a hymn on your lips or in your mind and heart, you will find it to be very therapeutic. Even singing in the shower is uplifting. If you have no musical talent you can appreciate a favorite kind of music, whether it is classical, Christian gospel, country western, or perhaps bluegrass. The music of stringed instruments such as the violin or harp can be very comforting and relaxing. These are all available on recordings which you can listen to during times of relaxation.

Another thing you could do is to get seriously involved in a hobby such as fishing and fly tying, photography, wood carving, bird watching, or rock collecting. There are organizations that provide fellowship and instruction in these activities. Women may find an interest in arts and crafts as well as some of the above activities.

In this computer age, there are challenging computer games that will exercise your thinking skills. Choose them carefully because there is also a lot of junk. Computer games tend to become addictive. A caution is to not get so involved in this that you devote too much time to it. It is important to maintain an active, well-balanced schedule of activities.

Keep in mind that physical ability and mental ability are interrelated, so if you are retired find some activities that will be both physically and mentally stimulating.

The attitude with which you face life is very important to your well-being. Maintaining an attitude that is lively, youthful, and forward-looking promotes longevity. People who think young and act young have an enthusiasm for life that keeps them going. They are always planning for the future like there will always be a tomorrow. They plant trees that will bear fruit in four to seven years, looking forward to enjoying the sweetness of the fruit. They keep involved in activities wherein they not only benefit but can be helpful to others. They learn and grow and stretch their minds. They look forward to fulfilling their desires with the attitude, "I can do this". In many ways, they become wise and apply their wisdom to enrich their lives and benefit humanity. These are people that will always be admired, respected, and looked up to. Ivis Meitler was a wonderful example of a centenarian who showed such enthusiasm. She got up early with plans for many things to do during the day. She thought young by associating with the youth in her church. She shared her musical talent daily with those in the retirement home where she lived. Although she lived in a retirement home, she was not merely warehoused to await death. She truly exhibited a wholesome zest for living that was stimulating to those with whom she associated. Rather than thinking of themselves as becoming old, weak, and useless, many seniors just zestfully keep going. This is the ideal way to approach longevity.

Finally, there are some supplements that can be taken to support brain function. Foremost among these is magnesium-L-threonate, which aids short-term memory, long-term memory, some learning functions, and moods. Taking folic acid, B6 and B12 helps to lower homocysteine. Eating oatmeal will help to regulate cholesterol. A Swanson product called Sytrinol can help you maintain a healthy cholesterol level. Ginkgo biloba aids the circulation of blood to the brain and acts as a blood thinner that will prevent blood clots. Do not take too much of this, though, as it may hinder clotting in the event of an injury. Taking vitamin K2 with ginkgo will help to counteract this problem. DMAE supports the neurotransmitters. One of the best products for cognitive support and nervous system nourishment is acetyl L- carnitine arginate. See the Appendix for supplement suggestions and suppliers.

Chapter Fourteen
Step 8: Medical Care

It is of utmost importance for every individual to know his own body and its physical needs. You must primarily be the person responsible for your own health care and decisions in that regard. To do this, you need to keep informed about current discoveries and changes in treatment methods. To facilitate this, you can subscribe to medical newsletters, bulletins, and journals. For aging people, the best publication is Life Extension (www. LifeExtension.com) Membership in Life Extension has many benefits, including low cost blood testing, access to and information about both alternative and prescription medications, and free advice. Be certain to keep careful records of your illnesses, doctor visits, and blood tests. You should have a physical examination at least once each year. When you keep your records, you can compare your status. Your physician can interpret blood test results for you so you can know how you are doing.

Each person should have a family physician that focuses on prevention as much as on treatment. If you are an aging person, it would be smart to have a physician who specializes in anti-aging medicine. This is a relatively new branch of the medical field, so unfortunately these physicians are few and far between. Another good choice would be an M.D. who also is educated on alternative medicine. In your reading, it would be a good idea for you to educate yourself about medical treatments including those used for alternative medicine.

Mainstream physicians are slow to accept alternative techniques, but the facts show that alternative medicine often succeeds better and with less expense than the traditional medical techniques of mainline doctors. That's why it's good to have a physician that is knowledgeable in both disciplines or, at least, is friendly enough to consider alternatives. But, remember, it's your body, and you should reserve the right to make your own medical decisions. That is why you need to educate yourself about the things that pertain to the problems you have or could potentially have one day. Do not make hasty decisions! Get a second or third opinion. Even then, be cautious. This author once cautioned a friend regarding a surgical procedure after he had a second opinion. I believed the procedure was too radical. The friend decided that the doctor should know what was best for him. Unfortunately, he died from the radical surgical procedure. Just a few years ago, a report in the Journal of the American Medical Association revealed that the leading cause of death was doctors. Doctors do make mistakes.[36] Consider also the number of deaths from new prescription medications that have caused some to be withdrawn from use.

Alternative practitioners are more willing to adopt new alternatives that are based on sound clinical tests, while other doctors may want to see more testing to be convinced. The medications that alternative doctors use are generally natural treatments that are safer than chemically devised prescription medications. They may or may not provide the desired results, but their use seldom has side effects, and they will not result in your death. When you get a prescription from your doctor, be sure to ask him how long the medication has been on the market, what the proven results are, and what the side effects are. You might also ask him about the cost of the drug or the procedure. When you take a prescription to the pharmacist be sure to ask about the details of the medication and the cost before having the prescription filled because you might choose not to use it.

A friend suffered an ocular migraine headache that caused temporary loss of sight in one eye. Leaving work, she went directly to an emergency room for diagnosis and treatment. Arriving there, she told the doctor of her history of ocular migraine problems. She was there about four hours while various tests were performed. At the end, the diagnosis remained as she had said in the beginning – an ocular migraine. She was given no treatment whatsoever. The costs for the procedures performed to satisfy that the doctor's diagnosis was accurate were $14,000.00. Insurance covers only about 80% of the cost. Many people turn to alternative medicine due to the increasing costs of traditional medical procedures.

Due to the prevalence of medical lawsuits, the medical profession often prescribes testing which may be excessive to confirm or disprove a diagnosis. This seems to be true especially when the patient has insurance. This in turn is the reason that the cost of medical insurance has drastically increased in recent years. It also partially accounts for the current downfall of the Medicare program.

It is unfortunate that, despite the large sums spent for health care in the United States, our success is not very great. On June 23, 2010, Health Day News reported the Washington, D.C. Commonwealth Fund's findings that, compared with six other industrialized nations, health care in the United States placed last in many respects. Also in 2010, the World Health Organization ranked the U.S. 31 out of 191 nations studied. Clearly, we have a long way to go in providing quality health care.
In the Journal of the American Medical Association, Barbara Starfield, MD., MPH of the Department of Health Policy and Management, and Johns Hopkins School of Hygiene and Public Health, talks about the deficiencies of U.S. medical care: Among her notes and comments are: "What has been found to be the major contributor to the excessively poor health of Americans is the health care system itself." She commented on deaths from unnecessary surgeries, medication errors in hospitals, other hospital errors, hospital acquired infections, adverse effects of prescribed medications which account for "230,000 – 284,000 deaths per year. These are the ones reported and do not include those not reported or adverse effects in going to private personal doctors including disability or discomfort."[37]

She continues as follows: "An estimate of adverse effects in going to private personal doctors and including adverse effects other than death concluded that between 4 percent and 18 percent of patient visits resulted in adverse effects in outpatient settings, resulting in 116 million extra physician visits, 77 million extra prescriptions, 17 million emergency department visits, 8 million hospitalizations, 3 million long-term admissions, 199,000 additional deaths (483,000 total medical deaths) and 77 billion in extra costs."[38] What this doctor is telling us is that the mainline medical establishment in the United States is the leading cause of deaths.

There are many excellent doctors in the U.S., and you want to be certain that yours is one of them. However, doctors are limited by their training and the policies of the establishment. That is why we say you must take responsibility for your health and your health care. Be informed and be cautious in making decisions, and don't fall into the pit of thinking that the doctor always knows best. Use good judgment in all of your medical decisions. Often when you refuse to follow a doctor's advice, you will be asked to sign a disclaimer which states that you chose not to follow the doctor's advice. This is intended to release the doctor from responsibility for the outcome.

Some mainline doctors continue to believe and stubbornly adhere to some things that have been proven to be untrue. One such instance is that they have believed that too much testosterone in elderly men causes prostate cancer. Now some doctors are proving that healthy testosterone levels in otherwise healthy individuals can actually cure BPH and can prevent prostate cancer. These doctors are using testosterone therapy to cure BPH and other results of testosterone deficiency.

Here is my testimony of how I came to appreciate alternative medicine practices. In my early mid-life I found myself needing to go to doctors frequently for various medical problems. It was frustrating because there never seemed to be a true cure. Much of the time, only the symptoms were being treated, and sometimes in the testing that was being done it seemed like I was being used as a "guinea pig" for the doctor's experiments.

On one occasion after I had a hernia surgery, I developed phlebitis. Several years later, I began to have stabbing pains in my chest. Sometimes they were so severe that I would go to my knees. The doctor could find no cause for this until finally he ordered a scan which revealed that I had a pulmonary embolism (a blood clot in my lung). The clot could not get through the lung tissue, and that was what caused the pain. It was supposed that the clot came from the leg in which I had phlebitis. This required a week of hospitalization for treatment.

A year or two later, I had another such occurrence. Then about one year after the second, I had another. They were getting more frequent when I had a fourth incidence of this at a very inconvenient time when I was visiting a relative far from my home. During a visit to my doctor following this occurrence, he suggested that the way to control the problem would be for me to take Coumadin for the rest of my life. Because taking Coumadin regularly requires frequent check-ups to regulate it and my work required many long trips traveling in a vehicle, I said, "I can't live like that." The doctor replied, "Well, then I have nothing else to offer you." This being the case I said, "Goodbye" and left his office.

I reasoned that when the Creator made human beings, He must have anticipated such problems and made provision for them. In His word, it says that the Lord "heals all your diseases" (Psalm 103:3). This is when I began my study of alternate medicine. I began to search for a solution for my problem. I found a book titled *"Earl Mindell's Vitamin Bible"* and read every word. The only helpful thing I found was that vitamin E was a blood conditioner. I could find nothing more to go on, so I decided to take 800 IUs of vitamin E daily. I later reduced the dosage to 400 IUs. In over 30 years, I have not had another incidence of a pulmonary embolism.

When I began to have kidney stones, I supplemented the doctor's treatment by looking for a cure. I discovered that vitamin B_6 and magnesium provided the cure. I have never had another stone since then. When I had persistent problems with urinary tract infections, the doctor had suggested drinking cranberry juice. I finally learned that D-Mannose was more effective than the juice and recently discovered that cranberry is most effective when taken as a softgel. One cranberry extract softgel has the value of 17 glasses of cranberry juice. The ingredients in D-Mannose and cranberry coat the lining of the bladder so that bacteria cannot stick and are flushed out.

Then I also learned that colloidal silver would kill not only bacteria but also viruses. When God created the earth and made silver, it was intended for more than money, jewelry, and industrial uses. Perhaps the most important use is as a powerful antimicrobial. Today, special clothing is made with silver fiber, Silver is used to make antimicrobial counter tops, and there are silver-impregnated band-aids to help prevent infection in cuts and burns. Collodial silver has many uses as an anti-infectant.

Some people are circumspect or even unwilling to use colloidal silver because they have heard of some who have misused it and had their skin turn blue. Properly used, it is entirely safe. Collodial silver was used by doctors prior to the advent of antibiotics, but many doctors today don't know what it is. You can get equipment and materials for making colloidal silver at home, and it is also readily available in health food stores. There are various kinds of colloidal silver. The quality is determined by the size of the silver particles; the finer the particles, the better. Look for at least 10ppm (parts per million). Mesosilver with 20ppm is an excellent product. We caution you to use it internally only when needed to counter a viral infection. In addition to taking it by mouth, you can spray it in the nostrils to cure a sinus infection or put a few drops in the ear to stop an ear infection. It can be safely used for many things in the home such as disinfecting your toothbrush, door knobs, and the blade on your can opener.

Inflammation and Pain: The Longevity Diet is intended to promote long life by preventing sickness and disease, but most everyone experiences some physical problems during life. One of the greatest health problems is chronic inflammation, so it is important to learn to recognize and control it. An inflammatory cascade occurs when injury or infection afflicts some part of the body. It manifests itself by heat, pain, redness, and perhaps swelling. Acute inflammation that ebbs and flows as needed indicates a well-balanced immune system, but chronic inflammation is a cry for help so that your white blood cells might carry away the inflammation. When they are not up to the task, the body can experience serious problems.

Inflammation can exist, quietly at first, in your internal organs. In the trachea and bronchial tubes, it can cause an asthma attack. In the kidneys, it can cause high blood pressure or kidney failure. It contributes to the onset of cancer, arthritis, asthma, allergies, and other diseases. Studies have shown that inflammation is responsible for frailty in aging seniors. Since there are not as many pain sensitive nerves in the internal organs, you may not notice pain to warn you of an impending problem. Constant low-grade inflammation in the internal organs has a nagging effect that can accelerate aging and cause an individual to be susceptible to disease. The medical profession does not have a definitive test to identify inflammation in the body. Testing blood levels of a pro-inflammatory marker, C-reactive protein, and the irritating amino acid homocysteine, are the best indicators known at present.

Inflammation caused by a nutritionally disagreeable diet may originate in the gastrointestinal tract. High carbohydrate, low protein diets are inflammatory while low carbohydrate diets tend to reduce inflammation. An individual may have a food allergy that could be the problem. Polyunsaturated vegetable oils like safflower oil, corn oil, and soy oil have an inflammatory influence, while olive oil is anti-inflammatory and contains disease fighting polyphenols. Following our Mediterranean-style diet will reduce the possibility of chronic inflammation.

Another serious cause of inflammation is emotional stress which raises the level of cortisol affecting insulin levels and metabolism and can create an inflammatory state. Stress may be afflicting a person subconsciously even though the person may not feel stressed. Environmental toxicity is still another form of stress that is caused by pollutants in the air we breathe, the water we drink, and various chemical contaminants that we come into contact with. Many of these contaminants are found in products used in the home and garden. It's important to use extreme caution when handling these chemical agents.

It is quite common today for people to use aspirin and other NSAIDS (non-steroidal anti-inflammatory drugs) to relieve inflammation. They are also used to relieve pain and fever. The most common NSAIDS available over-the-counter are ibuprofen (Motrin, Advil) and naproxen (Aleve). There are many more, such as Celebrex, that are available only by prescription. Tylenol (acetaminophen) has analgesic (pain relieving) and antipyretic (fever reducing) actions, but is not an NSAID. There are problems and adverse side effects that are associated with the use of these medications.

One of the problems with NSAIDS is that they can have a negative effect upon the immune system. For a person wanting to maintain a strong immune system, these drugs can counter that interest. Another problem is overuse which can cause drug-induced hepatitis. This can have a serious effect upon the liver and may lead to liver failure, which can be fatal. In this instance cessation of the medication and using burdock and/or milk thistle can detoxify the liver. Due to possible complications, doctors often require a blood test for liver function in persons using these medications.

With the exception of aspirin, NSAIDS may increase the risk of possibly fatal heart attacks and strokes in individuals who have underlying risk factors for these conditions. Prolonged use may increase a person's blood pressure. Including aspirin, there are possibly serious interactions with other drugs especially blood thinners like warfarin (Coumadin).

There are other, more natural ways of managing inflammation in persons who have a chronic inflammatory problem such as arthritis. Following a diet such as we recommend with The Longevity Diet is the first line of defense. This diet recommends using breads made with flour other than white flour, eliminating sugar and refined carbohydrates from the diet, and consuming plenty of fresh fruits, vegetables, and foods containing omega-3 oils. Inflammation can be further reduced with the use of turmeric, ginger, bromelain, or boswellia. There are two new products derived from turmeric that are now available; theracurmin, claims to be ten times stronger than turmeric; tetrahydrocurcuminoids (THCS) claims a broader spectrum and faster efficacy.

Acetaminophen (Tylenol) is a very common over-the-counter medication used for pain and inflammation. This is the preferred drug used in most hospitals. The use of this medication seems to be contrary to good medical practice. Statistics indicate over 450 deaths annually from its use. Other drugs have been withdrawn from the market for less cause, but so far the Food and Drug Administration has only seen fit, as of January 13, 2011, to limit the dosages to 325 mg. and to place warnings on the packaging. At least one-third of the cases of liver failure in the U.S. annually are attributed to acetaminophen. A portion of the FDA advice given to doctors states, "Severe liver injury, including cases of acute liver failure resulting in liver transplant and death, has been reported with the use of acetaminophen." Some scientists have urged removing this drug from use entirely. Despite the controversy regarding the use of this drug, it has not been withdrawn from the market because the negative effects are attributed to misuse. Many people do not adhere to the package directions, and this drug interacts badly with many other medications. It is also found in drug combinations. This will compound the amount of this drug a person gets if the individual is taking a drug combination plus additional acetaminophen. The bottom-line is that it is a very dangerous drug.

The good news is that there are some very effective and safe alternatives to these commonly used medications. The current star to counter inflammation is a naturally-occurring nutrient called astaxanthin (as-ta-zan-thin). This is an element that occurs in a microalgae found in the ocean. Since it is a fat soluable carotenoid, it possesses the typical orange xanthophyll pigment found in carrots. Its molecular structure gives it an exceedingly superior antioxidant capability. Not all antioxidants are also anti-inflammatory, but this one is.

This organism is eaten by salmon and causes the pink color of their flesh. It is also the reason that flamingos that are born with white plumage take on the pink coloring in their feathers. But, don't worry, taking it will not make you turn pink. This element also gives salmon the strength to swim upstream against powerful river currents and rapids and even leap waterfalls in their inland migrations. So, what can astaxanthin do for you?

There have been more than 9,300 studies, including in-vivo and in-vitro studies and clinical trials, to determine the effectiveness of astaxanthin. These studies consistently verify the therapeutic effectiveness of astaxanthin for a wide variety of applications. In the online newsletter, Natural News.com, (Tuesday, May, 08, 2008) Mike Adams, who takes this product himself, reported the following health benefits that have accrued to those using it:

- "Reduces proliferation of breast cancer tumor cells by 40%
- Protects the brain from dementia and Alzheimer's
- Greatly reduces inflammation and joint pain
- Reduces oxidative damage to your DNA by 40% (even at low doses)
- Greatly increases endurance, muscle recovery and workout performance
- Reduces the risk of cancer
- Causes cancer cells to commit suicide (apoptosis)
- Reduces the blood sugar level in diabetics and pre-diabetics
- Improves fertility while reducing the rate of stillborn deaths
- Promotes cardiovascular health, reduces C-Reactive Protein (CRP)
- Reduces or eliminates carpal tunnel syndrome
- Boosts immune function and helps the body resist infections
- Protects the stomach from ulcers and invasive bacteria
- Protects the kidneys from damage due to high blood sugar
- Generally improves sperm quality, motility and sperm count
- Prevents asthma by normalizing histamine levels
- Protects the body from highly oxidative foods like fried foods

- Greatly protects eye health, reduces cataracts and prevents UV damage to the eyes
- Makes skin look younger and functions as a natural internal sunscreen that prevents DNA damage and sunburn"[39]

These findings, confirmed by various sources, make astaxanthin seem like a miracle worker, and rightly so because it has such wide effectiveness for health issues in the body. Due to the extensive effects of inflammation in our bodies, it's likely that, as studies and usage of this nutrient continue, other benefits will be discovered. It is a supplement that is highly desirable to be added to an individual's daily regimen.

There are several advantages to astaxanthin that give it its superior capability. One of these is that, being fat-soluble, it can cross the blood-brain barrier, which makes it available to the brain, central nervous system, and the eyes. There it can relieve oxidative stress that affects many body functions. Another advantage is that it has as much as 500 times the antioxidant ability of vitamin E and 10 times the capacity of beta-carotene. Some laboratory tests rate its effectiveness as being superior to those of lutein, lycopene, and tocotrienols. It gives a powerful boost to the immune system functions all of which greatly protects the health of the body.

Astaxanthin is available in dosages of 4mg,8mg, 10mg and 12mg. The usual dose is 4mg, but Mike Adams says, "The more the better" and himself takes 16mg daily. It appears to be entirely safe with no known side effects. There are other sources of astaxanthin including yeast, crustaceans, and salmon but the natural *Haematococcus pluvialis* microalgae is far superior and is the preferred source. Because it is fat-soluble, it should be taken with foods containing fat such as omega-3 or perhaps just fish oil so that it will be absorbed into the body systems effectively.

While it might seem that we would not need any other anti-inflammatory medication, there is still another that is worthy of our consideration. Panitrol is an all natural alternative to Tylenol, Percocet, and other pain killers that are considered to be dangerous. This medication contains a combination of herbs that work synergistically to reduce swelling and inflammation of joints and blocks chronic pain receptors in the brain without disrupting the pain signals that warn you that a new injury has occurred.

Panitrol has passed a human clinical trial by Fenestra Research Labs, an organization known to be the world leader in wellness studies. This study involved 75 arthritis patients over a 30 day period. As soon as day 4 of the study, nearly half of the patients reported no pain. By day 14 of the study, 100% of the patients reported no pain at all. Amazing! This is solid evidence of the effectiveness of alternative medications.

The three primary symptoms of joint and muscle discomfort are pain, inflammation, and swelling. They are inter-related, and each can help make the symptom suite self-propagating. Panitrol mounts a three-pronged attack on these symptoms using properties from all five of its herbal extracts plus MSM (Methylsulfonyl Methanel) working synergistically and in concert. Its herbal components are juniper, goldenrod, dandelion, meadowsweet, and white willow.

While Panitrol is intended mainly to treat joint and muscle pain, it can be expected to give relief from any pain for which an individual would use Tylenol because some of its ingredients are natural aspirin-like compounds. These natural compounds have been found to give better relief than aspirin without any adverse side effects. Users of Panitrol testify that they have found relief from very old long-standing injuries that was much better than even prescription medications they had taken.

The makers of astaxanthin and Panitrol sometimes offer risk free 30 or 60 day trials of their medications. These can be found by checking their websites online.

With regard to pain there is yet another medication that is especially effective in the incidence of traumatic injury to the body or following a surgery. While we do not normally recommend homeopathy, there are some homeopathic remedies that really work well, and this is one of them. We are referring to arnica montana.

This comes in the form of a small tablet that is dissolved in the mouth, preferably under the tongue. In the event of a traumatic injury such as a sprain, concussion, bruising, shock, or strain from overexertion resulting in muscle soreness, arnica will work quickly to relieve the pain and bruising. Good results can be expected within 20 to 45 minutes. It can also be used to relieve night-time cramps. This makes arnica montana a good item to keep in your medicine cabinet or first aid kit.

This form of arnica should not be confused with the herbal form that is found in lotions or gels and is likewise effective for joint and muscle injuries. While one is taken internally, the other is always used externally. There are no known contraindications for arnica and no known side effects except that it should not be used too frequently as its effectiveness may diminish. Follow the dosage instructions on the container. One advantage of homeopathic remedies is that they are quite inexpensive.

A problem with many pain remedies is that they do not remedy the underlying cause of the pain, but instead merely treat the symptom. This is fine for immediate temporary relief, but it is much better to treat the cause whenever possible. Often the cause is inflammation or an injury. One medication that has been found useful for sprains, contusions, rheumatic pain, neuropathy, and other pains is DMSO. This is the abbreviation for *dimethyl sulfoxide*, which is a sulfur compound derived from the woody part of trees. One product containing DMSO is called Soothanol X2. Users testify to the effectiveness of this product, saying that just a couple of drops rubbed on the painful area relieves the pain in less than a minute. While this does not cure the cause, at least a person does not have to live with constant pain.

Bacterial Warfare: Many people are carrying a low-grade bacterial infection, usually in their intestinal tract, from which it circulates throughout the body. When it builds enough to overpower the immune system, the infection manifests itself as a urinary tract infection, a sinus infection, or some other type of infection. After an infection, some of the bacteria may linger in the sinus or urinary tract waiting for an opportunity to re-infect. It is important to take measures to eliminate, as much as possible, harmful types of bacteria from your body. You will never eliminate all of it, but you can minimize it.

In your intestinal tract, there are various kinds of bacteria. Some are good ones that are needed to aid the digestion process, but others are not good. There is a constant battle going on in your intestines between the good and the bad forms. When you take an antibiotic to eliminate an infection, it likely does what you want it to do, but it also harms the population of good bacteria in your intestines. This is an important downside to taking antibiotics and is one of the reasons some doctors are hesitant to prescribe them.

If you should visit a country where the water is not sanitary the bacteria, perhaps *e.coli*, may make you sick. This is commonly called Montezuma's Revenge. If you get such an infection, colloidal silver is an effective treatment. It is best to build resistance in advance to ward off such infections, though, and the best way to do that is to take probiotics. These include *acidophilus, bifidobacterium lactis, lactobacillus casei, lactobacillus acidophilus,* and *bifidobacterium bifidum.* These strains of good bacteria overpower the bad bacteria in the intestinal tract. They are made more effective by also taking a prebiotic, FOS (brand name Nutra Flora), which nourishes the probiotics. Probiotics are obtained in The Longevity Diet when you eat yogurt; however, you build a more effective population of probiotics in the intestines by taking them as supplements. These probiotic supplements are also an effective treatment for a bacterial infection but will take some time to become effective.

There are natural antibiotics that one can use to defeat an infection. These include vitamin C, zinc, green tea, and garlic. Those on The Longevity Diet are likely already taking most of these, but when an infection occurs, larger doses than are used as a preventive are necessary. There are several ways of taking garlic. You may include garlic cloves or minced garlic in your diet, but with these you risk having it on your breath. A good alternative is Kyolic garlic, which is a supplement specially formulated to avoid this problem.

When there are harmful bacteria in the urinary tract causing an infection, it is helpful to take measures to cause them to be washed from the body. These bacteria have hair-like fimbriae that help them to adhere to the walls of the urinary tract where they propagate and infect. Cranberry juice helps prevent this adherence. Cranberry gel cap supplements are much better than the juice, and D-Mannose is also very effective for this purpose. When using these products, the bacteria are flushed out with the urine.

There are also products that help to overcome bacteria in the intestinal tract that cause diarrhea. Imodium A-D is the most effective drug to stop diarrhea; however, it causes the organisms causing the problem to remain in the intestines for a longer time. A good alternative treatment is kaolin and pectin (Kaopectate), which absorbs bacteria and passes it through the gut, or bismuth subsalicylate (Pepto-Bismol), which neutralizes the poisons created by bacteria. Both of these are available in liquid or tablet form. For the treatment of bowel irregularity, the use of psyllium powder is highly recommended. It only needs to be taken at night before retiring. It can be mixed with six ounces of juice. Psyllium is also available as Metamucil (brand) cookies, which are convenient when traveling.

Helicobacter is a bacteria that causes infection in the stomach and can cause ulcers to form. Coriander, which is also protective against salmonella, is helpful to kill the bacteria, as are horseradish and garlic.

Diabetes has become the seventh largest health problem in the United States today, and its prevalence continues to increase. This is caused by excessive glucose (sugar) in the diet and the insufficiency of insulin. As this problem has serious consequences including possible amputation, blindness and death, it is important to control and seek to cure it. None of the medications prescribed by doctors are a cure, and some are not helpful. Therefore, other means are necessary to combat this problem. Controlling the diet is the primary means of therapy. Losing weight is important, and The Longevity Diet generally is helpful with some modification. It is essential to eliminate most sugar and fat from the diet. Eating beans on a regular basis, perhaps even daily, has been found to be effective, as is eating apples. An "apple a day" is aptly applied here. Whole grains are also important. Sweeteners should have zero calories.

When managing a diabetic diet, it is important to eliminate saturated and processed fats. Eating salmon and other cold water fish is recommended, as also is the extra–virgin olive oil according to The Longevity Diet plan. Eat a moderate amount of protein, but avoid consuming high-fat dairy products on a regular basis. Again, focus on eating plant foods; vegetables, legumes, and nuts are best according to The Longevity Diet plan. A high-complex-carbohydrate diet with high fiber content will help to maintain blood sugar levels.

The minerals vanadium and chromium (chromium picolinate) are good supplements to promote insulin sensitivity. The suggested dose of vanadium is 100 mg and for chromium picolinate it is 200 mg daily which should be taken with meals. An ingredient found in your kitchen which is also helpful for insulin sensitivity is cinnamon (if it is the pure unadulterated product). You can sprinkle it on toast and oatmeal, but it is most effective in the extract form available in capsules. A good dosage would be 300 mg daily.

To complete the program, be sure to drink plenty of green tea and exercise as recommended. A person who judiciously follows this plan, along with other suggestions found elsewhere in this book regarding sweeteners and glycemic indexes and loads, may manage, improve upon, or perhaps even cure diabetes. A final word here is that if diabetes has progressed to the extent that it affects the legs and feet, it may be wise to consider hyperbaric oxygen therapy before deciding upon amputation.

Heart Disease: Whereas in earlier times heart disease was not common, in our present culture it has become the number one killer. This is mostly due to our changing lifestyles and a diet that includes many prepared foods. Those who follow The Longevity Diet should have little difficulty with heart disease, but if you have not been following this lifestyle plan you may already be in danger of heart problems. Some of the early symptoms of heart problems are chest pain, shortness of breath, an irregular or faster heartbeat, weakness, fatigue, lethargy, daytime sleepiness, nausea, sweating, lightheadedness, and dizziness. If you have any of these symptoms without a reasonable explanation, a physical exam to determine the cause would be in order.

Cholesterol is a contributing factor to plaque in the arteries which restricts the flow of blood. Diet and supplements can help to control cholesterol and plaque, However, the best thing a person can do for heart health is to keep active. There are two forms of exercise that should be used for optimum conditioning. The first is aerobic exercise. Regardless of what you may have read elsewhere, it is important to exercise daily during all seasons of the year. Aerobic exercise includes activities such as walking, running, bicycle riding, and swimming. For heart health, it is important that exercise sessions last one full hour. That may seem like a tall order, but consider that in previous times when people had little heart disease or in areas today such as the Hunza Valley where there is a small incidence of heart disease, the people walk many miles each day. But that is a tall order when a person is not accustomed to it. So it is suggested that a person start with 20 or 30 minutes daily and work up to the one hour goal. Discipline is important to meet your goal, and to assist with discipline it is helpful to have another person committed to walk with you. That way each keeps the other accountable.

The one hour session is important because "what you may not know is that your body has what's called a 'collateral circulatory system', a microscopic network of blood vessels that ordinarily remain closed. With sustained physical activity – such as a daily hour-long walk – these vessels open and become enlarged, forming an alternate network to bring blood to your heart. When these vessels open, it causes a "second wind" feeling of prolonged aerobic exercise.'[40]

The second form of exercise that is needed is resistance or strength training. This is especially important for men over 50 years of age because their diminishing hormones result in likewise diminishing strength and muscle mass which is the cause of flabbiness. Actually, men of any age who tend to be sedentary can benefit from resistance exercise. This form of exercise involves things such as weight training and exercises using barbells or various specialized equipment found in gyms.

The stresses caused by using tobacco products, drinking alcohol, and eating excess fatty or sweet foods lead to problems for heart health as do emotional stress, aggression, financial problems, and other sickness.

In addition to following The Longevity Diet there are some supplements that are especially helpful to maintaining heart health. Some of the most important supplements are antioxidants, which we have discussed previously. Garlic is quite commonly used to prevent cardiovascular problems. It is best used with ginkgo, magnesium, and calcium to help control blood pressure. Studies have shown that garlic also lowers total cholesterol. You can definitely lower cholesterol and triglycerides by adding a good amount of omega-3 to your diet. This is available in some foods but also in fish oil and flax oil. The omega-3 has blood thinning properties. Vitamin E is valuable since it coats the platelets of the blood and helps to prevent blood clots from forming. Coenzyme Q10 has several helpful applications to heart problems. If angina is indicated, CoQ10 is helpful. It is also helpful for arrhythmia along with magnesium, L-carnitine, and potassium. Higher dosages of CoQ10 can have a dramatic effect on congestive heart failure and it has also been found helpful in cardiomyopathy.

Note: Glucose Spikes that occur following a meal have been found to be very dangerous for seniors and anyone who has diabetes or cardiovascular problems. These spikes considerably increase the risks of retinal damage, cardiovascular disease, diabetes, and cancer. Life

Extension has reported studies that reveal the serious dangers of these spikes. "After every meal, these sudden surges in blood sugar damage delicate blood vessels in your brain, heart, kidneys, and eyes, as well as accelerate the aging of cells and tissues throughout the body. . . Without controlling fasting and postprandial sugar spikes, the stage is set for accelerated aging and a series of degenerative diseases."[41]

Scientists have discovered a green coffee bean extract that is helpful in controlling sugar spikes. Being aware of the extensive dangers of these surges makes it essential for individuals at risk to control their calorie intake to effectively reduce these dangerous glucose elevations.

Healing Panaceas: A healing panacea is a substance that will seemingly miraculously, act as a cure for a wide variety of ailments. These are usually inexpensive compared to traditional healing therapies. The Health Sciences Institute has compiled an encyclopedia, "Miracles From the Vault" which is invaluable to those desiring to use alternative medical treatments (see resources in the appendix). This volume is available to its members with their membership fee.

You may recall from our discussion of various cultures that the people of Hunza, who drink water called "glacial milk" flowing from the ice-blue high mountain glaciers, have very few heart problems or other diseases. Scientific studies have indicated that the glacial water contains nano-colloidal particles of minerals, especially silica, and a large amount of negatively-ionized hydrogen which causes the glacial water to have an enhanced alkaline content. The exceptional health of the people is attributed to drinking a good amount of this water. The people of other regions such as Mongolia, Ecuador, and Peru who also live in similar high mountain areas and drink glacial water likewise enjoy the anomaly of the people of Hunza.

Of course, we cannot all move to one of these mountain areas to benefit from this water, so scientists have searched for ways to duplicate the quality of the glacial water. The Japanese were the first to invent a machine that was capable of producing enhanced hydrogen alkaline water. They put these machines in their hospitals to aid in the recuperation of their patients. Similar machines are now available world-wide. These machines typically purify the water and increase the hydrogen content, yielding purified alkaline water. You will find sources for these in the resource section of this book.

It must be noted that hydrogen is the energy source of the universe, beginning with the sun and including all life on the earth. Water is two parts hydrogen and one part oxygen. An individual can live longer without food than without water. If an individual could eat only pure raw organic vegetables and fruit, the individual would be charged with abundant energy and good health. Enzymes in the body release hydrogen from the food we eat. This hydrogen is thus burned by oxygen, and the burning produces energy. This explains the benefit of eating raw vegetables and fruit as called for in The Longevity Diet. The well-being of the universe is attributed to an abundant supply of hydrogen.

There are many benefits attributed to drinking as little as two glasses of hydrogen-charged alkaline water daily. These include the removal of toxins from the body, reducing pain, repairing cellular damage, improved mobility, general improvement of health, increasing energy levels, and reversing the aging process.

The neutral pH of pure water is 6. The pH of hydrogen alkaline water is 9 or more. This higher pH factor can be obtained in several ways. One can add a few drops of food grade hydrogen peroxide to a glass of water and then drink the water; however, some doctors warn that this might be corrosive to the arteries. Similarly, a teaspoon of bicarbonate of soda added to an eight ounce glass of water with stirring will increase the pH of the water from 6 to 9. Some dentists advise their patients to rinse the mouth nightly before retiring with one tablespoonful of food grade hydrogen peroxide for dental health reasons If the rinse is held in the mouth, especially under the tongue, for a few minutes, some of the hydrogen will be absorbed into the bloodstream.

Another, perhaps more desirable, means of duplicating the benefits of "glacial milk" was invented by Patrick Flanagan, who did a careful study of samples of water from Hunza. He discovered that the minerals were carrying negative ionized hydrogen. He also discovered the electron in every bodily chemical reaction that is responsible for giving life. He was able to devise a means of trapping an abundance of negative ionized hydrogen ions in silica spheres where they would remain until added to water at which time they would be released. The product of his discovery is called Microhydrin. His product contains not only the regular electron but also the life giving electron. When the product is consumed, it has an amazing ability to neutralize free radicals.

Microhydrin is a nutrient that produces noticeable results in as little as 20 minutes. Individuals have noticed increased energy, sharper vision, and brighter colors. It is not toxic and will not interfere with any drug or therapy. It has been found to detoxify the body by chelating heavy metals to eliminate them from the body. At the time of this writing little information seems to be available from scientific studies of Microhydrin except for those conducted by the inventor.

Hydrogen Peroxide: Recognizing that hydrogen is the essential energy source of the universe we must not underestimate the enormous potential of hydrogen peroxide to enable healing of cancer and virtually all diseases. This solution consisting of the molecular structure $H2O2$ has one more molecule of oxygen than water which makes all the difference in the world. Oxygen engenders life and promotes healing. This natural oxygenating substance has the potential to revitalize and rejuvenate healthy cells, thereby creating vibrant energy and well-being.

Otto Heinrich Warburg was a German physiologist and medical doctor. His love for cellular research earned him three nominations for the Nobel Prize. He was the Director of the Kaiser-Wilhelm Institute of Cell Physiology where he studied the respiration of cells. From his studies he concluded, "The prime cause of cancer is the replacement of the respiration of oxygen in normal body cells by a fermentation of sugar."[42] Warburg further concluded that most disease is caused by insufficient levels of oxygen in the body. Peroxide works by increasing tissue oxygen levels.

Actually peroxide is essential for life and is created in the body but not in sufficient quantity for all healing purposes. Most strains of harmful bacteria cannot survive in the presence of oxygen.

Hydrogen peroxide is helpful in the treatment of a host of diseases including cancer, arthritis, diabetes type II, asthma, prostatitis, yeast infections, Parkinson's Disease, bacterial infections, and viral infections. The only peroxide that should be used for internal purposes is 35% food grade.

Peroxide can be administered orally or intravenously. The use of peroxide is not without some risk, including death, if not administered properly. It is best to do this under the direction of a doctor trained in its use. To find a doctor contact the International Bio-oxidative Medicine Foundation, P.O. Box 13205, Oklahoma City, OK 73113 or phone at (405)478-4266. There are books available that explain the protocol in much more detail than can be included here. For these see the resources at the back of this book.

Suggested Procedure: The solution must be diluted to a 3.5% solution. Undiluted solution should be kept in a freezer. Diluted solution may be refrigerated. A 3.5% solution can be made quite easily by first pouring 1 ounce of 35% H2O2 into a glass measuring cup. Then, with stirring, add 11 ounces of distilled water. The mixture will be 12 ounces of 3.5% H2O2. (Do not use chlorinated water to dilute the peroxide).

35% Food Grade H2O2 must be handled carefully. Direct contact will burn the skin. Should you have an accident flush well with water and then apply aloe gelly to the burn. One of the most convenient methods of dispensing the solution is with a small glass eyedropper. Mix the drops into 6 to 8 ounces of distilled water, fruit juice, or even aloe vera juice or gel.

"The program outlined is only a suggestion, but is based on years of experience, and reports from thousands of users. Those who choose to go at a slower pace can expect to progress more slowly. Individuals who have had transplants should not undertake an H2O2 program. It stimulates the immune system and could possibly cause rejection of the organ.

On day one take three drops three times per day. Increase the dosage by one drop per day up to day eight. Then increase by two drops up to day sixteen. The maintenance dose in most situations is to taper off gradually as follows: 25 drops once every other day for one week; then 25 drops once every third day for two weeks; then 25 drops once every fourth day for three weeks. **It is important to take hydrogen peroxide only on an empty stomach.**

If you are not taking vitamin E and acidophilus, I recommend starting them before starting the H2O2 protocol.

If you experience a healing crisis; fatigue, diarrhea, headaches, skin eruptions, cold or flu-like symptoms, or nausea do not discontinue using the peroxide as it is due to body cleansing. By continuing the program, toxins will clear the body sooner and this healing crisis will pass rather quickly."[43]

Aloe Vera: Many years ago this author first experienced the healing wonders of aloe when he discovered that aloe gelly would miraculously heal eczema better than the prescribed cortisone ointment he was using. Aloe vera comes in the form of juice, gel, gelly, and as a powder in capsules.

All aloe is not the same. In addition to the various forms, there are inner leaf and whole leaf varieties. An individual choosing an aloe purchase must be careful because some products have other substances added and are not pure aloe. These combinations should be avoided. When making a purchase look for the seal of the independent International Aloe Science Council (IASC) that validates the aloe content and purity.

Aloe gelly is very effective applied topically to first and second degree burns, minor cuts, or lesions in the skin, including chapped hands, an incision following surgery, scrapes or puncture wounds. It will also aid the healing of scars. In addition to its healing properties many people like to use it as a moisturizer under make-up, or to apply after shaving. It is often found in skin lotions, howbeit, in very small amounts. It is a wise idea to keep a tube of 99% aloe vera gelly in the first aid kit or the medicine cabinet for emergencies. A lady who had a pressure cooker explode on her chest and face said that, because she quickly applied aloe to the scalds, she healed quickly without any scarring.

Aloe juice, or gel can be used internally and most often, about two ounces is added to another juice. In these forms it supports stomach acidity, and may be healing to peptic ulcers. It also aids digestion, enhances antioxidant support, and gives a boost to the immune system.

Whole leaf aloe powder, in capsules, has a great number of applications, perhaps, most notably for pain relief. The impressive list of applications include several forms of cancer including, lymphoma; metabolic disorders, including, kidney disease, and type 2 diabetes; neurological disorders, including Parkinson's, and dementia; bone, muscular and skeletal diseases including arthritis; cardiovascular diseases, including atherosclerosis, and stroke, plus it is useful for irritable bowels, and other intestinal problems.[44]

The miracle working benefits of aloe are due to its polysaccharide "agents of life" which have the ability to pass through the digestive tract to the cells of the body without being destroyed by stomach acids or digestive enzymes. There are over 300 nutrients in aloe including amino acids, minerals, enzymes, sterols, vitamins, lignin, salicylic acid, and saponins. These work in concert to create harmony in the body. [45]

The inner leaf aloe powder in capsules is principally used to counter constipation. It is very effective for this purpose, but should not be taken continuously for more than ten days because the body could come to depend upon it.

Another panacea is **Miracle Mineral Solution (MMS).** This is sometimes called Master Mineral Solution. Although it has been widely used in Europe, it is little known in the United States. This product is exciting because users actually report miraculous results. Cancer patients in the fourth stage of the disease and in hospice care have been completely cured in only a few weeks.

MMS was coincidentally discovered by Jim Humble when he was leading an exploratory expedition in the Amazon jungle. Two of the men in his group came down with malaria. Neither medical help nor medication was available. However, he did have a bottle of stabilized oxygen, a liquid solution of sodium chlorite used for purifying water. He reasoned that if this solution would kill bacteria in water it might also purify the blood of his sick men. After ingesting the solution, both men were miraculously cured and ready to go within four hours. Due to this amazing experience, he continued to experiment and developed the product which has cured over 75,000 documented cases of malaria plus a host of other ailments.

Based upon thousands of testimonials, MMS has been found to effectively treat and cure most ailments that are caused by a pathogen. Pathogens are micro-organisms including mold, viruses, bacteria, and fungi that can cause disease in their host. They can live in our bodies for years without being detected and escape allopathic procedures. When something occurs to weaken the immune system, these pathogens seize the opportunity to attack. These biological agents cause disease in the gastro-intestinal system (colitis, Chrohn's disease), the urinary system (kidney and bladder infections), the respiratory system (colds, flu, pneumonia), the cardiovascular system (anemia, hypertension), the neurosensory system (hearing loss, visual problems, migraines, cognitive dysfunction), the musculoskeletal system (joint problems, mobility), and in the skin (rashes, dermatitis, edema). There are more possible applications than are indicated here.

In her "MMS Miracle Book, A Journal of Protocols & Testimonies", Tammy Olsen relates, "It was not until the testimonies from thousands of people came through to me that I began to realize how the magnitude of this discovery could actually change the world and ultimately bring new hope to many people who had lost all hope." [46] If you are interested in using MMS, it is suggested that you get a copy of Tammy Olsen's book.

One form of MMS requires mixing with a citric acid activator just prior to adding water or juice and drinking it. A newer formula does not require mixing. The product is normally consumed two or three times daily. There are various protocols for its use, but it is not our purpose to explain them here. Rather our purpose is to inform our readers of this discovery and its possibilities.

The Longevity Therapy: Recognizing that oxygen engenders life, we want our readers to be aware of an experimental therapy that has great potential for bodily healing, regeneration, and rejuvenation. Anything that you can do to effectively saturate all the cells of your body with oxygen will markedly improve your health. You would do this exercise early in the day when your body is well rested. You may precede the therapy with a very light breakfast such as a slice or two of multigrain bread spread with Smart Balance Omega 3,and also, perhaps a piece of fruit.

First, with a large (12 oz.) cup of hot green tea, take your antioxidants, fish oil or flaxseed oil, astaxanthin, vitamin E, CoQ10, Alpha Lipoic Acid (R-Fraction) along with ginkgo biloba, and acetyl L-carnitine arginate (this form is essential to the therapy) to aid circulation across the blood brain barrier. This sets the nutritional stage of the therapy.

Second, relax for 30-45 minutes; this might work well as you might have a devotional time including Bible reading, prayer and meditation. You may like to use a devotional guide for this exercise. This sets the mental and spiritual stage of the therapy.

Third: This stage is a combination of physical exercise and breathing. For this step, you will need to wear an oxygen mask to insure that you are breathing only pure oxygen. With the mask in place and the oxygen flow adjusted, you will walk on your treadmill or peddle your stationary bicycle at the fastest speed that you can maintain for at least 30 minutes. After that time, you may take a brief rest (not more than 5 minutes) while continuing to breathe pure oxygen. If you have both of the machines indicated, you may then switch to the other one, and, again, at the fastest pace that you can maintain, continue for another 30 minutes, at which time you will have completed the session for that day. It is preferable to repeat the therapy three to five days each week. The more frequently you do the therapy, the sooner and better you will realize the benefits. As you continue the therapy, you will find it easier to do. Note: A good flow rate of oxygen is suggested. You may need to adjust the flow of oxygen as you exercise, so place the tank near enough that you will be able to do this without interrupting your exercise. If the flow rate is too low, you may fatigue too quickly. Adjust the flow rate according to how you feel. It is advisable to be accompanied by another person for this exercise period. To avoid boredom you may want to watch TV or read a book or magazine while on your machine.

If you don't own these machines, this therapy can be done at a gym or fitness center. Another option is to mount a small oxygen tank on a cart and go walking outdoors or in a mall. Malls usually are not very crowded early in the day. If you are walking, it is essential that you keep up the fastest pace that you can sustain.

Managing medical costs: In these times when the cost of medical treatment is increasing and not affordable for many, and with the uncertainty of Obamacare, or a similar program, which will create health care rationing for seniors and death counseling for those with disabling and potentially fatal diseases, it is important for individuals to educate themselves about ways that they can effectively care for and treat themselves at home in the event of a health problem. We have tried to show that this is possible. There are likely to be cutbacks in Medicare and Medicaid, and private insurance plans are becoming very expensive. We cannot count on the government or an insurance company to take care of us.

An alternative to health insurance is membership in a health care sharing plan, otherwise known as a health letter plan. These plans, whereby members help each other to pay medical expenses, are less costly than insurance. A member who has a health care need receives health care treatment from a provider of his choice. He sends the bills to the plan administrator, who verifies that the need meets the plan guidelines. Then, in a monthly newsletter, certain members are directed to send their monthly share directly to a particular member to cover the cost of his need. In this manner, members help each other to meet medical expenses. These plans usually don't pay for preventive costs such as physical exams, so members need to have a savings plan to cover this type of expense. The plans are usually Christian based. Their advertisements can be found in Christian publications and conservative news magazines. Also refer to the reference section of this book.

Another option to help pay medical expenses is a medical discount plan. Individuals pay a monthly fee for this service, and health providers give a considerable discount to the patient. These plans are helpful to those who cannot afford the high rates of medical insurance.

Disclaimer: All medical information contained in this book is presented for educational purposes only. Please keep in mind that alternative treatments are usually primarily used as preventives, although they have been found in many circumstances to be healing. Success using these suggestions is not guaranteed. Some have been cured of cancer. Hyperbaric therapy has helped many stroke victims, and some have found other cures for various ailments. What works for one individual may not work for another. Except for personal experiences cited, we have only reported the results of our research. We have touched on some core problems, but keep in mind that a pain reliever is not a cure; it only relieves the symptom. What you want is a cure. That is why we recommend that you have a doctor who will partner with you as you use these alternative treatments. Without such professional help, you are on your own to use your best judgment.

Chapter Fifteen
Step 9: Financial Security

Living long and living well means that an individual will need to have sufficient finances to provide for needs during this extended lifespan following retirement. A person who retires at age 65 and lives to be a centenarian will need sufficient resources to carry him through 35 years of life. These are years that can require considerable expense with limited income. Assuming that the household consists of a husband and wife, there will be two to provide for. If a couple have both had incomes, their combined pension plans may ease the retirement budget.

During an individual's working years, it is important to plan for the retirement years. There are four avenues of preparing for retirement. The first of these is personal savings. All too often this is neglected, not possible, or limited due to the income level and the cost of living. When it is possible to provide some savings, the interest rates of banks is so low that the savings will not accrue much interest. It is better to invest personal savings in an annuity that will provide a good payout during retirement. The second avenue is Social Security (SS). Unfortunately, the SS system is depleted, or nearly so; therefore the future of SS is uncertain. The third resource to prepare for retirement is a pension plan. While these are provided for those working for a government agency and some corporations, they are not made available to all workers. Social Security and pensions are not intended to fully provide for all of the needs of the retiree. It is important for the retiree to be able to provide for much of his own needs. Many people use investments, which is the fourth avenue, to round out their retirement needs.

It used to be that the average person could invest in some common stock of a good company and earn a good profit, but, over the years, stock market investing has evolved into a more sophisticated system involving much more risk. It is wise to heed the warning, "Past performance is not a guarantee of future gains". Indeed, during the downturns of the stock market, many have lost much, or even all, of their retirement savings, so beware of the greed of Wall Street. Moreover, with the deteriorating condition of the American economy it is unwise to invest in common stocks as their value can go down to zero very quickly even though the investment may be in a good company.

It is an indisputable fact attested to by the best economists that the American economy is currently headed for failure. There are many reasons for this. One is the inflation that has occurred since World War II. In 1945, wages were low, but so was the cost of living. A loaf of bread could be purchased for 5 or 10 cents. A cup of coffee was five cents. The gas bill for a home using natural gas for cooking and water heating was less than ten dollars per month, and regular gasoline was twenty-five cents per gallon. Let's assume a $20.00 purchase of groceries in 1945 compared to 2011. The cost for the same groceries in 2011 would be $250.80, and the inflation rate is 1154.0%. Inflation has gone up and down over the years, but the trend is that it is going up. As inflation goes, so goes the cost of production and the cost of living.

At this time, there are many people who are jobless due to layoffs and the new people entering the job market. The jobless rate has been increasing rapidly since 2008. The federal government manipulates the jobless rate in their method of computing it, so it is said to be about 10%. According to a very reliable reporting firm, Technometrica Market Intelligence, the unemployment rate for the second week in July 2011 was 28.6%. The unemployment rate during the Great Depression was said to be 25%. If the truth were known and admitted, we are already in the greatest depression this nation has ever known, and it will only get worse.

The worst factor responsible for our economic condition is that our government spending has been out of control, and their spending has led to a tremendous debt. At this time, the debt is said to be over $17.3 trillion. However, nobody seems to know the actual amount of debt. Estimates of the true debt range from 75 to 114 trillion dollars. Since 2008 when President Obama was elected as President, the national debt has increased faster than ever by trillions. The generosity of the government has outdone itself. The Social Security Program at one time was very solvent, but Congress took huge sums from this entitlement fund to pay other debts, so that today the future of Social Security is dubious. The Medicare program is also out of control, costing enormously more than the amount taken in each year.

Years ago, the Treasury Department began borrowing money from other countries to pay our national debt, and much was borrowed just to pay the interest on the debt. No person or nation can continue to borrow to pay their debts without coming to a point where they can no longer continue to do that. The United States is at the point of no return today because no other nation wants to lend more to us. Those who hold our debts are trying to divest themselves of it through trade or whatever means possible. The result is that the U.S. has become the greatest debtor nation in the world and has exhausted its credit rating. Another result that further lowers our status is that the International Monetary Fund has recommended that U.S. currency no longer be used as the reserve currency for international trade. Russia and China have already made agreements that forego the American dollar. Arab nations are following suit. In some nations, tourists have some difficulty paying their expenses with American dollars. The American dollar is no longer considered to be of much value since America is so far in debt.

Up until 1933, the American monetary system had gold to back up the value of its currency. At that time, President Franklin Roosevelt recalled all of the gold coins and exchanged them for paper currency, so the United States was no longer on the gold standard with gold to back up its currency. In 1963, President Nixon drove the final nail in the coffin, making our currency totally fiat currency backed only by the faith and credit of the government of the United States. After that, our dollar bills no longer stated "Silver Certificate" under George Washington's picture. Silver dollars still being used in trade in some places were taken out of circulation. The United States is rapidly approaching the time when it will default on its debt, and there will be no faith and credit for the U.S. monetary system. This is estimated to occur by 2015.

What will happen then? Nobody seems to know for sure because there doesn't seem to be any plan for that contingency. The United

States currency that has been decreasing in value for many years may not be worth a Confederate Dollar used by the Southern states during the confederacy. If there is any value to the dollar, it will be greatly diminished. There will be considerable inflation due to this devaluation. Some speculate double-digit inflation, though others doubt that. Can you imagine a loaf of bread costing $20.00 or the price of gasoline making it unaffordable to drive a vehicle very far? It is likely that we will also have to pay higher taxes to reestablish our ability to build our nation. Due to the imminent seriousness of the problem, it behooves every citizen to be prepared. It may take ten to twenty years to grow out of this travesty.

A further consideration is that if the currency becomes valueless, how could a person purchase or pay for anything? The government may need some time to reestablish a monetary system. Therefore, everyone should prepare by accumulating essential food items such as flour, beans, rice, pastas, canned, frozen or dried fruits and vegetables sufficient to last for at least six months to one year. Those who live in a rural area where they can produce food items will be most fortunate. Even on an acreage or large lot a person can produce a lot of food. Garden seeds are another thing to accumulate; keeping at least enough for a year or two ahead on hand is a good idea.

One thing that we must always keep in mind is that no matter how desperate the situation may become, the potential for survival and happiness is not in things, but in people, our families, friends, and neighbors. It will be important to love God, and to love one another and stick together through all of the hard times, sharing whatever we have with one another. A person can be poor and needy and still be satisfied by cleaving to loved ones.

Another thing that you should have is firearms and ammunition. Although we don't advocate eating red meat on The Longevity Diet, it may become necessary, and wild game, properly prepared, is better for you than the meat of some domestic animals. You may need firearms to get some game for food or to protect yourself and your family from desperate people who will try to rob, steal, and, if necessary, kill to survive. Another possibility is that an enemy nation may seek to take over our nation if it perceives weakness providing an opportunity.

Investment Opportunities for Future Security. One thing that we are told is that what is coming in the future will be worse than the great depression of the 1930's. The stock market may crash, and banks may fail, but there are some investments that are certain to endure and provide income until a new monetary system is established.

Good blue chip corporations are not going to disappear when the crash occurs, but you must choose very carefully before investing, and **do not buy or hold any common stocks**. If in your timing you see that the crash is near and you can invest in options you could short (buy a put option) the S&P Index, but that too could become worthless in U.S. dollars. A better plan would be to invest in certain Exchange Traded Funds (ETF). One fund currently doing well is the Powershares Db US $ Index (ticker symbol UDN). This investment tracks the yield performance, subject to fees and expenses, of the Deutsche Bank-US Dollar Futures Index. The fund does well because the US dollar is falling against the German Mark. This fund is designed to replicate the performance of the dollar against the Euro, Japanese Yen, British Pound Sterling, Canadian Dollar, Swedish Krona, and the Swiss Franc. Remember that with such investments timing is very important, and follow your investments on Yahoo Finance or through your brokerage. Careful timing is essential to know when to get out of these investments and put your proceeds in a safe place.

Perhaps a still better idea would be to get out of American dollars completely. Especially, don't hold cash because it may become worthless. You could invest in certain investments, say perhaps, in Canadian or Australian currency. Both Canada and Australia are English speaking countries, and their rate of exchange is favorable at the time of this writing. Exchange your dollars to their currency when investing. An annuity in one of these countries could be a good investment. As it pays out, its currency likely will be worth more than whatever currency the U.S. is using. Foreign investments can be made through the Toronto Stock Exchange or through international banks such as Evergreen Bank. Be sure to check out the taxes and fees that these countries will levy on your earnings.

At the present time, many believe that the best income investment in the U.S is **preferred stocks**. These stocks differ from common stocks in some very important ways. The most important is that they represent ownership in a company. Their value does not depend on the rise and fall of the stock market. Their purchase price is their par value, and their value may rise or fall a little, but they will not become worthless as common stocks can become. These stocks pay a stated dividend, usually quarterly. This dividend payment must, by law, be paid before earnings can accrue to common stocks. If the preferred stock is rated as cumulative but the company cannot pay the dividend, it must pay it in the future whenever funds become available. This makes preferred stocks one of the very safest investment vehicles. In the scenario we are considering, when the U.S. monetary system fails, you will still own a share of the company, and when a new monetary system is established, you will resume receiving income that will be cumulative to account for any lost dividend payments.

When considering a preferred stock purchase, you will want to choose a good company that will withstand the fall of the economy. The wisest choice is a company that deals in something that the citizenry cannot do without. At the top of the list is food, and very close behind it is energy. Considering our enormous dependence upon electric utilities, just imagine trying to get along without this power source. In rebuilding our economy, technology will also be very important.

To find a good company that has preferred stocks you can go to an online brokerage site or to Yahoo Finance. Find a good company by studying its charts, To learn if the company issues preferred stocks, go to QuantumOnline.com. There you can do a quick search using the common stock symbol. Next, by clicking where it says, "Find All Related Securities For (symbol)", you will discover all of the securities that the company or its subsidiaries have available.

Now let's consider an example. We know that electric utilities are a needed business. We have found that the Southern Company based in Atlanta, GA has been cited as the World's Most Admired Electric and Gas Utility by Fortune Magazine in 2011. You can't do much better than that! We find that a subsidiary, Alabama Power Co., has preferred stocks available. We choose 5.83% Class A Cumulative Preferred Stock available on the New York Stock Exchange with the symbol ALP-O. We have learned from this site that the par value is $25 per share and that it can be recalled at the same price plus accrued dividends. The income from the stock will be a 5.83% dividend that will be paid quarterly. This is money you can count on, whereas with a common stock the value can go up or down to zero. Another important feature of this investment is that the dividends are eligible for the 15% tax rate. This stock can be purchased using an online brokerage just the same as common stocks but using the appropriate ticker symbol.

It would not be wise to put all of your eggs in one basket regardless of how good an investment may be, so we will look at the next safe investment vehicle. Another sector that consistently pays good dividends is **Master Limited Partnerships (MLP)**. An MLP is a publically traded limited partnership. Again, your shares provide ownership in the partnership, however, they are officially referred to as units rather than shares. These businesses usually own and operate pipelines that transport commodities such as oil, natural gas, and gasoline. The larger the holdings and distribution area of the company, the better its position for profits. Another plus is that the energy demand will continue to rise over the foreseeable future.

These MLP's are required to pay out most of their cash flow to their shareholders. As the income depends upon product volume, their distributions are quite stable. The average yield is 7%, but it can be considerably higher. The profits from these investments derive from growth in face value and from income of the dividends paid. While it is possible that the face value could go to zero, it is highly unlikely. The mixture of income safety and growth makes MLP's desirable for your investment portfolio. Another desirable feature is the tax advantages they provide. As a partnership, they are not subject to corporate income taxes. However, due to the way they are taxed, they are not suitable for investing in an IRA or a 401 account. They are best suited for an individual brokerage account. Should the holder become deceased, they are an excellent inheritance due to the way they are valued in this instance.

MLP's can be found by going to QuantumOnline.com, which provides a list of them that you can sort through. Let's look at an example of an MLP. Atlas Pipeline Partners LP (ticker symbol APL) has a present face value of about $32.89. APL owns and operates five active gas processing plants and approximately 8,600 miles of active interstate gas pipelines. They also own other interests. Atlas Energy. LP, is an MLP that is the

General Partner of APL. Atlas owns an interest in over 8,500 producing natural gas and oil wells. APL was paying dividends of about 0.95 per share when it reached a high point on 03/07/2007. Following the crash in 2008, it plunged to a low face value of 2.95, but as early as March 2, 2009 it paid a dividend of 0.66. Since then it has been making a great comeback. Although dividends have varied, the last dividend paid was 0.40, giving a yield of 4.80%. Just today as this was being written, the next dividend was approved at 0.47, which is a 17.5% increase above the last dividend. This demonstrates the resiliency and potential for this MLP to move toward its previous high position. The holder of 100 units of APL will receive a dividend payment of $47 in August 2011. One thousand units would net a dividend payment of $470. The face value of 1000 units would be about $32,800. If the dividends are reinvested rather than withdrawn, the value of the investment will compound.

While there is potential risk of loss with an MLP, there will always be income from dividend payments the same as with preferred stocks. The difference is that the dividends may not be cumulative. If you would like some expert help in analyzing these types of investments, consider subscribing to an excellent advisory newsletter called High-Yield Investing. See the resource section of this book.

Precious Metals; Gold, Silver, Etc.: Maybe it was just because they glitter, but since the earliest time, when gold and silver were discovered, value was attributed to precious metals. People fascinated with these metals learned to make jewelry with which they adorned themselves. The attractiveness of the adornments gave value to the metals. They also gave status to the one so adorned. Thus gold, silver, and other metals such as platinum came to be regarded as precious metals.

With intrinsic value attributed to them, these metals came to the forefront to be used to make coins which were used for money; thus a monetary system based on precious metals had something tangible as its foundation.

When America was founded, the citizens first used coins of other nations such as Spain, France, and England, but then the United States established a monetary system using coins minted of gold, silver, and other metals right here in America.

Because coins were heavy and it was impractical to carry many in the pocket. Paper money was created that was a certificate representing a specified amount of gold or silver for which the certificate could be redeemed if the bearer so desired.

Since the United States went off the gold standard, its paper money has been fiat currency, sanctioned by the federal government, based solely upon the faith and credit of the government. Due to unwise budgeting and spending practices, often without regard for the financial ability to do so, enormous debt has accumulated that has nearly completely eroded this "good faith and credit" of the United States. Nations such as China that have loaned huge sums of money to the U.S. have no assurance of ever being repaid. When the U.S. can no longer borrow to pay the interest on its debt, there will be no alternative but to default, on its debt which will void the "good faith and credit" promise.

Gold and silver, which are indestructible, always have value because they are something tangible; that is, it has real value. Owning physical gold is the oldest way in the world to possess something of value. Although gold has been used for money, it is not money but rather an asset that represents a certain monetary value. That is to say, there has to be a value system upon which to attribute value.

The value of gold in U.S. dollars has recently escalated to $1600 per ounce and, at this writing, ranges between $1200 and 1600 per ounce. Some economists and gold dealers speculate that, as the value of the dollar falls, the value of gold will increase but that the increase will be in deflated dollars. The saving grace in this scenario is that gold is recognized worldwide as a desirable commodity. India and China are especially interested in acquiring gold. When the U.S. defaults and its money is seriously devalued, it will have serious repercussions worldwide, but the monetary systems of other nations will continue to place a value upon gold, silver, and other commodities.

As the U.S. seeks to recover, it will need to reestablish a monetary system that should be based on something tangible. Gold is the most likely candidate. In March of 2011, the legislature of the State of Utah enacted a law, signed by Gov. Gary Herbert, which reestablishes gold and silver coins issued by the U.S. Mint as legal currency rather than an asset in the State of Utah. Of course, the coins can be used only at face value, and gold is valued so much higher than paper dollars that nobody will be using them as money at this time. An establishment bank, J.P. Morgan, announced in February of 2011 that they would accept gold as collateral for loans as an alternative to the U.S. dollar. Stock exchanges in the U.S. and Europe have started accepting gold for some trades. Previously, the U.S. valued the dollar as 1/135 of an ounce of gold. Going back on the gold standard will require the U.S. to establish a new valuation.

Among the nations, of the world the United States possess far more gold than any other nation. Should the U.S. default on its debt, those who hold physical gold in any form may be most fortunate because they will possess the standard. The U.S. has a legal provision allowing for the recall of gold being held by the citizenry. This was done in 1933 but has not been done since then. The need to increase our national store of gold may be the impetus for a recall. By the current law, United States gold coins dated before 1933 will be exempt from recall. These are considered collectibles, so such coins are the most desirable to preserve your wealth. Any gold surrendered to the government should be compensated with the new currency at the established valuation.

Now that we have established the desirability of owning physical gold, we will look at some of the best ways to secure a supply to preserve your wealth and future financial security.

The most obvious way to obtain gold (or other precious metals) is to purchase it from a gold dealer. There are many local dealers in cities across the nation. Don't overlook this possibility. The advantages are that you can examine the gold before purchasing and then take immediate possession. There are also several reputable large nationwide coin dealers that offer a wide selection of coins of various precious metals from many nations around the world. If they are reputable, they will send you coins on approval, but they will not ship coins until they safely have your payment in their account. Be certain that you are dealing with a reputable dealer. Coins that are collectible are usually graded coins certified by one of the two recognized grading services, which are PCGS or NGC. The highest grade of coins is MS70, but any coin graded MS is a good coin. Grading is one way of having assurance of quality and value. You may be able to get a better selection and pricing from these national dealers that usually issues a catalog and advertises widely. Caution: It is generally not wise to let someone else store your gold for you. They may charge for the service. The gold may or may not actually be there, and it is most readily available to you if it's in your possession. It is also not advisable to store your gold in a bank deposit box. If the bank should fail, your deposits would not be available.

The next option is to invest in a gold **Exchange Traded Fund (ETF).** Note that although these are stock funds, some of them are acceptable because they hold physical gold for every dollar invested. You can even request to have your gold shipped to you if you desire to withdraw your investment. One advantage of an ETF is that you have more latitude in the amount of money you invest. If you purchase a coin, you will need to pay the full price upfront but with an ETF you can invest a lesser amount and then add to it as you desire and allow your investment to grow. Caution: There are specific risks in this type of investing. You should carefully research any investment to be sure it is right for you.

The safest, most acceptable type of ETF for investing in gold or other precious metals is a gold bullion ETF. These investments are trust accounts backed by actual physical gold that is purchased and held in storage as individuals invest. There are others that do not hold physical gold and are therefore not desirable as safe investments. An individual can invest in these funds by buying one or more shares of stock through a stock broker. Some online brokerages offer the lowest fees for this service. There are three funds that we have considered:

1. SPDR Gold Trust Symbol, GLD: New York Stock Exchange (NYSE) Arca. This is the most popular of these funds, and it holds the most gold. The price is based upon 1/10 of the value of one troy ounce of gold. The price varies daily according to the market. At this writing with the value of gold slightly over $1600 the share price is $157.32

2. Ishares Comex Gold Trust, Symbol, IAU: NYSE Arca. This fund is different because its price is based upon 1/100 of a troy ounce of gold. This makes it less expensive to get started buying gold. On this same date as the GLD share price was $157.32, the value of one share of IAU was $15.77. Keep in mind that you are buying less gold with each share.

3. ETFS Physical Swiss Gold Trust, Symbol SGOL: NYSE Arca. This fund bases its share price on the value of 1/10 of an ounce of gold.

On the same date, it was $160.36. The main difference with this fund is that the physical gold is stored in a depository in Zurich, Switzerland. This may or may not be a desirable advantage. At least it will be out of reach of the U.S. Government should they desire to recall gold from the citizens.

The safest way in the world to own gold is said to be **Perth Gold Certificates**. The Perth Gold Certificate Program (PMCP) is sponsored by the Perth Mint in Western Australia. Silver and platinum can also be purchased through this program. These certificates can be purchased from dealers in the United States. The initial purchase must be at least $10,000 after which you can add to the investment in increments of at least $5,000. There is a fee, usually 2.25% to buy the certificate and 1.25% to sell it.

The mint is owned by the Government of Western Australia, which is very secure. By law, it must own the precious metal before it can make a sale. The metals are stored at the Mint, which is located on the western coast of Australia. All of the precious metals are insured by Lloyd's of London at the Mint's expense. This is the only way to have your gold insured unless you personally purchase the insurance. Your holdings are also guaranteed by the Government of Western Australia, which has a AAA credit rating. Should the U.S. economy collapse and dollars become worthless, you will still own whatever amount of gold you purchase, although you may not know its value until a valid monetary system is established. Nothing is a safer asset to own than gold, and it is safest at the Perth Mint.

Note that much that has been said about gold can apply also to silver. Many people cannot afford to invest in gold, but could purchase or invest in silver. This metal is considered by some to be a better choice, because silver has many uses besides being used as money. It has many industrial uses, and is used for jewelry. There are also medical applications such as colloidal silver. Coins with smaller values (nickels, dimes and, quarters) are available for trading when our monetary system collapses. Some predict that the value of silver will outpace the value of gold, in which event, it will be the wiser choice.

America's wealthiest families have a "secret" way that they have used to preserve and grow their wealth even in times when the economy is down. They buy and hold rare coins that have considerable value. These are referred to as **numismatic coins** or coins with numismatic value. They are generally rare collectible coins that are in good condition. Under present U.S. law, these coins are safe from confiscation by the government. The value of some of these coins is millions of dollars, but most coins have much less value. Interested persons can establish a trading account with a rare coin wholesaler with a minimum investment of $50,000. The wholesaler will hold your coins and offer them for sale privately, at auctions and at shows, to secure a profit for you. If you own coins that you don't want to trade, you can hold them privately or in a depository. These dealers also offer a free coin evaluation service to determine the potential value of your coin.

Often these rare coin wholesalers will offer coins that are rare due not to age but to their content or mintage. Recently one dealer, Rare Coin Wholesalers, offered a U.S coin of recent mintage. This is the 2008 one ounce American Platinum Eagle with a $100 face value. This is the highest face value of any coin. Platinum is more rare than gold and presently is undervalued, so the potential is there for considerable gain. Among older coins, currently a 1918-s Buffalo Nickel has a value of $19,500. The value of other Buffalo Nickels is as high as $89,500, but there are many with lesser values. The bottom-line with coins is that they are worth whatever a buyer is willing to pay for them. Don't think that coin collecting and dealing is only for the ultra-wealthy. As you are involved, you may stumble upon something that someone will pay a lot of money to own.

Warning: Many people have their retirement savings invested in a 401 (k) or an IRA account. The current federal administration has been considering taking over these government-authorized accounts as a means of reducing the national debt. One proposal has been to confiscate the accounts and offer a government annuity that would pay the individual in small increments. Protect yourself from this possibility by investing most of your assets in other places. Also be aware that when the government defaults any treasury notes that you are holding will become worthless. China doesn't want them, so why should you?

A final word about investing. When an investment is going up in value, we are pleased, but we should set a figure at which we will be satisfied. Some think to let the investment's value ride up and up as long as possible. With stocks, in particular, the trend may suddenly turn, causing you to lose principle. Learn to control you psychological impulses. A person must learn not to be greedy. Enough is enough! Learn to be satisfied with a reasonable profit. The inverse is also true when trading a falling investment with a put. Circumstances may change, causing the trend to turn. In these uncertain times, be aware that in an economical crisis you must have time to reinvest or withdraw your earnings safely.

Poor Man's Survival Techniques: You may never have been able to save and invest or perhaps you have already lost your savings due to the economic downfalls since 2000. It is not shameful to be poor. Jesus, who was, Himself, dependent upon others, honored the poor. Be of good courage and use your resourcefulness, trusting the Lord to bless your efforts. Where there is a will, there is a way.

Bartering was used prominently before there was money, and directly exchanging goods and services has continued to be a useful practice up to the present time. You are likely not alone. You can network with others in your community to help one another. When you have the opportunity, strive to be self-sufficient. Plan for where you will live, what you will eat, and how you will heat and cool your home. Share your resources of food, material things, and labor with others, and don't be reluctant to receive help from them. Others who are more fortunate will be willing to help you and will find a blessing in doing that. Don't deny them that blessing by being too proud to receive their help.

Although you may be cash poor, you still probably have some resources. Perhaps you own valuables that another would buy from you, such as antiques, firearms, jewelry, coins, stamps, or other collectibles. You can clean these things to make them presentable and offer them on eBay, at a local flea market, or on Craig's List. Although these things may have sentimental value, don't allow yourself to drown in your sentiment. They are of real value only as you derive the value from them to preserve your livelihood. Remember, you can't take them with you.

You are your own best resource. You are a person of value, and you may have much to offer to others. There are organizations that employ caregivers. If you have love in your heart and some physical ability, you could be a caregiver. Surely there is someone who would appreciate you and be willing to recompense you for your tender loving care. If there is no organization to place you, advertise yourself by word of mouth or in classified ads.

Some do well with a home-based business. There are many of these to choose from, but beware of the requirements to get started, and don't be lured by exaggerated claims of potential income. Study the opportunity carefully, perhaps checking out the company's reputation with the Better Business Bureau. You may be able to use your resourcefulness to develop your own home-based business.

One man that I knew when I was a youth, told me that he survived the Great Depression by making hammer handles and selling them house to house for 25 cents. If you have a skill, such as landscaping, carpentry, seamstress or quilting you can use it to good advantage. Others have survived difficult times by doing odd jobs or by collecting scrap to sell. You may even be able to live off the land. In the spring, some folks in my hometown used to go along digging dandelion greens from lawns. They are actually tasty! George Vreling, as indicated in his biography, was blessed to be able to buy a farm where he did well. The seller may be willing to let you buy real estate with a note if you are short of cash, but prove yourself worthy. Some have lived on and managed a farm for an absentee landlord. Maybe you can make a deal with a bank. Today, banks own many foreclosed homes, some of which require repairs and maintenance. Even in the worst of times the Lord blesses those who help themselves while trusting in Him.

> *"Better is a little with righteousness, than vast revenues without justice."*
>
> *Proverbs 16:31*

Chapter Sixteen
Step 10: The Will to Live

There are many stories of a person who was terminally ill who held onto life until some loved one was able to arrive so that they could be together at the end. The will to live can be very powerful. The appreciation for life with the desire and will to live has been innate in humans from their creation.

Throughout the ages, there have been countless stories of individuals who have been caught-up in death, defying circumstances and have survived against overwhelming odds. The only explanation for their survival is that the will to live kept them going. Such are the stories of some biblical heroes, of American pioneers like the seven Sager children who pushed on alone to Oregon after their parents died along the way, of Corrie ten Boom who survived the German holocaust, of Jake DeShazer, who survived as a Japanese prisoner of war during World War II, and of those in recent times who have survived being buried under rubble for an excessive time following an earthquake. The will to live exists to give each one of us hope to survive the circumstances of life. With faith in God, we know with all of our being that God will make a way. Every bit of our energy is applied to hold onto life.

Dr. Norman Vincent Peale wrote and spoke much about the power of positive thinking. It was his belief that by applying positive thinking techniques a person could achieve any goals in life. He wrote, "Once you establish your goals, how do you reach them? By the application of a twin principle: to *will* and to *believe*. Will power is the process by which you utilize an enormous force that is within you. Believing is the process by which you surrender yourself to the power of God. So "to will" means to bring out your personal power; "to believe" means to bring out God's power. And, if you really begin to practice the principle, your achievements can be astonishing [47].

Peale's belief, based upon numerous experiences of his own and others, was that a person could enter into a relationship with God whereby the person could **believe and will** himself to health, to wealth, and to succeed over many circumstances of life if the principles of positive thinking found in scripture were consistently applied in the person's life.

The will to live, when firmly set and rooted in faith in God, firmly entrenches mind over matter so that the cosmic power of the universe, by which all the universe was created, assists an individual to overcome overwhelming odds. The will to live can be your best asset in living long and living well. Keep in mind that "I can do all things through Christ who strengthens me" (Philippians 4:13); remember also the true teaching of Christ, "The things which are impossible with men are possible with God" (Luke 18:27).

The one who sets his will must be obedient to follow the leading of the Holy Spirit, Who prompts every cell of one's being in the direction in which he must proceed. Spiritual and intellectual insights that stimulate strength and endurance are brought about by obedience to the Spirit dwelling within.

Most who succeed in living long and liking it are endued within to seek the ultimate, deepest, and most spiritually rewarding things of life. They succeed in their inner being to be all that the Creator created them to be.

To have the will to live means that we must focus on life rather than on death. To focus on death is to engender a spirit of fear. Such fear places a negative stress upon an individual's life that is defeating. Faith in the future casts out all fear and focuses positive energy toward achieving the "desires of your heart" (Psalm 37:4).

As we focus on life, we keep thinking about what we will do in our tomorrows. We plant flowers and anticipate their lovely blooms. As we garden this year, we are already planning and looking forward to an even better garden next year. We plant fruit trees that may not bear fruit for several years visualizing the enjoyment of their sweet fruit. Visualizing is one of the techniques by which we embrace the future. So, as we live this life, we just focus (visualize) on living so that we can live with happy, productive years.

The greatest joy of life is to have the assurance that the end of this earthly existence will simply be a transition or a relocation of the soul to our heavenly home. We were made for life – not for just a few years on this earth, but for eternity.

While we measure our present life in years lived, eternal life has nothing to do with time and everything to do with the ultimate quality of existence. It is an existence that is totally removed from all of the struggles of our present life to an existence in which the joys of this life are superseded immeasurably. This present life with its difficulties and trials will culminate in a heavenly inheritance, the gift of God, which consists of "all things" (Revelation 21:7). This gift includes all that you could desire and more than you can imagine. Those who have died and then been brought back to life tell of a glorious place where they momentarily experienced great joy in the presence of the Lord and saw loved ones who had gone before.

John, the apostle of love, shared his vision of our heavenly existence (Revelation 21:3-8). He envisioned it as a place where "God will wipe away every tear from their eyes; there will be no more death, nor sorrow, nor crying; and there shall be no more pain, for the former things have passed away" (v. 4).

As we focus and plan for our future, we must make preparations for the continuation of life in heaven. We will do this by desiring and building in our lives the characteristics that will make us suitable for life in heaven. The one thing that God cannot do is allow any sin in heaven. The supreme moment of this life is when you make the final decision, once and for all, that sin will no longer live in you – that it will die completely - not merely be constrained, or suppressed, or countered, but crucified so that you are dead to sin such that it no longer has any place in you (Galatians 2:20).

Death to sin brings the satisfaction of knowing that you have done well and God will give you your heavenly inheritance as a child of God, (Rev.21:7). The sin of pride will be changed to humility. The sins of selfishness and greed will be overcome by sharing, generosity, and hospitality. Because of the love of God reigning supreme in our lives, we will find fulfillment in being and doing all that we can for others with a true servant heart that does not look for some return benefit, but only delights in giving and sharing as we are able to help others in need.

The will to live will engender in our hearts the love of God and a peace that passes understanding. Motivated by love, we have the will to live long and live well. With the will to live, we care for our bodies, minds, and souls that God has given us in such a manner that we can be all that God desired and intended us to be when He created us.

What matters now is that we will have the desire and the will for the gift of eternal life so that we will place our complete trust and apply our life force toward the goal of receiving our supreme gift.

It's Satan's desire to cause us to deviate from our great potential; he wants to steal the gift that was inherent in our creation. That gift possesses the cosmic power of God to keep us going against all odds. Our hope in God and our human will are the determining factors in our ability to achieve our full potential.

Willpower is meaningless without the ability to choose. Choice requires an alternative. The consequential alternative given is death (Genesis 2:17). As we walk through this life, we will face many choices. These choices will be between self and Christlikeness. Disciplining ourselves to choose Christ instead of ourselves is actually learning to overcome our selfish nature. The more we choose to let go of self, the more we take on the nature of Christ and secure the potential power of life that is our unique gift.

Dr. Peale has written, "You and I possess the power to *choose*. . . you can *choose* to be happy. If you are driven by fear, *choose* to be courageous. . . If you are weak and sick, *choose* to be well. . . In Deuteronomy 30:19, it says, 'Choose life that thou . . . may live.' So you have an immense power, the power to choose."[48]

The fact that you are reading this book is evidence that you value life – your inherent God-given gift. Should you be one who chooses to believe the premise made herein, you are on solid ground whether or not the premise is true. Should you risk not believing the premise, you have made your choice to forfeit the possibility of truth and to accept the risk of a regrettable demise. Choosing wisely will guarantee the rewards of life.

Roy L. Smith told the story of "an elderly man, past eighty years of age, who was lunching with a young friend who was impressed by the octogenarian's vigor, alertness, and apparent youthfulness. The younger man knew that the older one was doing a full day's work in his profession every day, and putting many a younger man to shame with his achievements. Furthermore the younger man was impressed by his friend's outlook and plans for the future. Finally, in a burst of confidence and an appropriate apology he said, "Sir, if you would forgive the question, I would like to ask how old you are? "The old gentleman turned merry eyes upon his questioner, pilloried him for a moment in pretended sternness, and then said: "My son, my age is none of my business."

"The number of years we live is unimportant. The kind of years we live is all that counts. Eternal life denotes a quality of life as well as quantity of life and any man can have it.

The man of eighty years can be very young; the man of forty can be very old. A man's age is actually none of his business. His work, his duty, his responsibilities – these are the things which make life. And these enjoy the priority of our concern.

According to our Christian interpretation of life, we have a work to do as long as we have strength and time in which to do it. No man is demobilized by his birthdays. To think about one's age is to become a bondsman to it."[49]

Conclusion

The purpose of this book has been to present our research on the various aspects of life that contribute to living long and living well. As you have seen, The Longevity Diet involves much more than the food that you eat. Indeed, life is much more than food, and living well involves much more than owning a luxury home or vehicle. For some people, living long is largely a matter of inheriting the right genes, but, as we have shown, a person can enhance the quantity and quality of one's life by adopting the lifestyle we have presented herein. Living well greatly improves upon the prospect of a long life.

While we have sought to show the physical aspects that contribute to a long healthy life and the dietary means of sustaining a healthy body, we have moreover sought to reveal the significance of an individual's philosophy of life, faith, and also the social and emotional interactions that contribute to the wholeness and wholesomeness of life. As has been indicated, if there is any one aspect of a person's life that is most important, it would have to be spirituality for it best encompasses the essential part of life from conception throughout the years of life until the person passes from this world. As an individual who values life, giving serious attention to the spiritual aspect of life, and considering one's body as the temple of the Holy Spirit, while using this book as a guide, all of the other aspects of life will tend to be drawn together to create wholeness of life. This in turn will add length of days to a person's lifetime.

I trust that by reading this book the reader has acquired information that will stimulate and enable living long and living well as so many others, including many centenarians, have managed to do. Their numbers are increasing, so you have a good opportunity to succeed. If you do succeed, the purpose of presenting this work has been achieved.

Jesus said, *"The thief's purpose is to steal, kill and destroy. My purpose is to give life in all its fullness,"* (John 10:10 NLT).

For God so loved the world that He gave His only begotten Son, that whoever believes in Him should not perish but have everlasting life, (John 3:16).

Living Meaningfully

by this same author, is the perfect companion volume for those who want the most from life. Here you will discover the rule of life, the essence of life, and the pathway to victorious living. You will find answers to life's tough questions. With this guide you will truly be able to settle into the values of life that make life truly worth living.

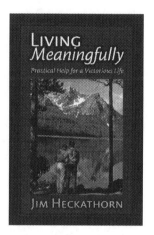

Acclaimed by readers as
"inspiring and insightful" (Tessa)
Written in *"a warm and caring way"* (Jim F.).

Senior adult readers commented,
"It provides Scriptural and practical solutions"
(Jerald);
"I could hardly put it down until I read the last page.
(Charles)
"Very interesting... I read it through a couple times"
(Thelma).

Every reader who values life and desires the ultimate satisfaction from living will benefit from reading this book.

Special Offer for readers of How to Live Long and Like It... $10.00 plus $5.50 for priority shipping. Mail your order with check or Money Order to: Morningstar Meadow, P.O. Box 136, Elk City, ID 83525

Appendix

Resources and References

Air Purification Systems:

Fresh air is essential to our well being. If you live in an environment that contains mold, mildew, or other pollutants, one of these systems will be helpful. There are special heating system filters and attachments and also stand alone units. One of the best is Eden Pure, Call 1-800-370-8249, www.edenpureair.com

Alkaline Water Purification Systems:

The people of Hunza drink "glacial milk", which is pure water with a high hydrogen content which is highly antioxidant. Pure water is essential, and if you desire a high hydrogen content some of the best systems are

Emco Tech Co. (Jupiter Science)
Athena – top performing machine.
Elita – world's only non-electric machine, is not reverse osmosis so preserves all minerals. www.ionmicrowater
DetoxifyNow.com, www.kagen-aqua.com

Bible Study and Devotional Aids:

RBC Ministries, Our Daily Bread, Grand Rapids, MI 49501-2222, www.rbc.org
www.discoveryseries.org
Supernatural Healing and Phenomena, www.sidroth.com, 1-800-548-1918

Coin Dealers; Gold and Silver:

Preferred Customer Club, www.govmint.com, 1-800-946-6526
Rare Coin Wholesalers, www.RareCoinWholesalers.com
Discover the potential of numismatics, 1-800-347-3250
Universal Coin and Bullion, 1-800-459-2646, www.universalcoin.com
United States Money Reserve; 1-866-441-4653, www.usmoneyreserve.com
First Fidelity Reserve, 1-800-336-1630, firstfidelityreserve.com

Financial Information and Advice:

Carla Pasternak's High-Yield Investing, 1-800-796-8025, www.high-yieldinvesting.com
The 12% Letter, Dan Ferris, Editor, 1-888-261-2693, Stansberryresearch.com
Retirement Millionaire, Dr. David Eifrig Jr. MD, MBA, 1-888-261-2693
www.stansberryresearch.com/products
Lee Bellinger's Independent Living, 1-877-371-1807

Financial Services – Stock Broker:

Scottrade (Online services nationwide), www.scottrade.com

Food Products – Flour & Grains:

Joseph's Grainery (organic grain), 1-206-853-7961, www.josephsgrainery.com
Bob's Red Mill, 1-800-553-2258, www.bobsredmill.com
The Teff Company, 1-888-822-2221, www.teffco.com
Premium Gold Flax Products, Grain and All-Purpose Flour (gluten free), 1-866-570-1234

Health Information:

Life Extension Foundation: Keep up to date with health science and services. Life Extension members receive the magazine, quality cost effective blood testing, advice, and quality vitamins and supplements plus excellent pharmacy service.

Life Extension Foundation, 1-800-544-4440, www.lifeextension.com

There are many health newsletters. We recommend:

Health Sciences Institute (Senior memberships are discounted and include their health encyclopedia, *Miracles from the Vault*, (203) 699-4416, www.hsibaltimore.com

Nutrition and Healing, Dr. Jonathan V. Wright, M.D., www.wrightnewsletter.com

Health and Healing, Dr. Julian Whitaker, M.D.,(800) 539-8219, www.drwhitaker.com

Health Radar, Get Healthy No Matter What Your Age, A Newsmax Publication, 1-800-485-4350, healthradar@newsmax,com

Second Opinion, The independent thinker's guide to health and wellness, 1-800-791-3445

The Blaylock Wellness Report, Living a Long, Healthy Life, Dr. Russell L. Blaylock, M.D., 1-800-485-4350, wellnessreport@newsmax.com

Alternatives For the Health-Conscious Individual, Dr. David G. Williams, M.D., 1-800-527-3044, custsvc@drdavidwilliams.com

Diseases Don't Just Happen, (video) Lorraine Day, M.D., 1-800-574-2437, Rockford Press, P.O. Box 8, Thousand Palms, CA 92276

Dr. Barry Gordon, M.D. Brooklyn, NY, Online videos on testosterone, www.thehiddendisease.com

Discover Hormone Optimization

AAG Health Clinics (20 locations nationwide), AAGHEALTH.Com, 1-888-387-0999

Juicing:

Raw Vegetable Juices, N.W. Walker, D. Sci., Pyramid Books, 919 Third Avenue, New York, NY 10022

Medical Insurance Alternatives:

Samaritan Ministries, Christian Families Helping Each Other, 1-888-268-4377, www.samaritanministries.org

Medi-Share, Christian Care Medical Sharing. (This plan also supplements Medicare), 1-800-722-5623, www.medi-share.org

Vitamin and Supplement Suppliers; Anti-aging Products; Medical Supplies; Prostate Solutions:

Master Mineral Solution (MMS), Keavey's Corner, (863) 824 – 7575, www.keavyscorner.com

Mesosilver Colloidal Silver, Colloids for Life, LLC, 800-390-5839, www.colloidsforlife.com

Puritan's Pride, Vitamins, supplements, aromatherapy, massage oils, and more., 1-800-645-1030, www.puritan.com,

Swanson Health Products, Complete line of products including those used in homeopathy., 1-800-437-4148, www.swansonvitamins.com

Scriptures, A line of vitamins, supplements, beauty aids, and Bible studies. Also an employment opportunity. Reference code 66445 when contacting or ordering. 1-877-850-5156, www.scrip.com

Unikey Health, Ultra H-3(HGH Secretagogue),, 1-800-888-4353, www.unikeyhealth.com

Quality Health Blends, Inc, Alpha–HGH, 1-800-717-5145, www.ALPHA-HGH.com

Hampshire Labs Inc, GHR Growth Hormone Releaser, 1-800-279-5517

CTG Clinical Testosterone Gel 1.92%, 1-888-462-1797, www.ctg192.com

Bio-Renew Nutrient, Energy Greens and Other Nutrition Products, Institute For Vibrant Living, P.0. Box 3840, Camp Verde, AZ 86322, 1-800-218-1379, www.takebiorenew.com/save

The One Minute Cure to Healing Virtually All Diseases, By Madison Cavanaugh, Think-Outside the Book Publishing, LLC, 8484 Wilshire Blvd., Suite 760, Beverly Hills, CA 90211

The Magic of Hydrogen Peroxide, James Direct, 500 S. Prospect Ave., Box 980, Hartville, OH 44632,

Aloe Vera Products, Nature City, 900 S. Rogers Circle, Boca Raton, FL 33487, 1-800-651-3066, www.naturecity.com/save

BioStem,The stem cell generator, 1-888-379-0563

StemCell-Maxum Natural Rejuvenation (reverses aging; offers no-risk guarantee), www.HealthyHabitsWeb.com, 1-800-604-6766

Reverse Memory Loss

Rebuild Memory and Brain Power, NeurosPlus www.GetNeuroPlus. Com, 1-877-419-7681

ProceraAVH (Free trial, Satisfaction Guaranteed), Boosts Memory and Mood, Brain Research Labs, Westbrook, ME 04092, 1-800-916-4868, www.brainresearchlabs.com

Macular Rejuvenation

Healthy Vision Complete, True Health, www.truehealth.com, 1-800-746-4513

Home Study Courses

The Great Courses, 1-800-832-2412, www.buygreatcourses.com

Seniors Organizations
(offer insurance and discount medical service programs)

Association of Mature American Citizens (AMAC), Bohemia, NY 11716, 1-888-262-2006, www.amac.us

Work at Home Guaranteed Supplemental Income

Morningstar Meadow, Elk City, ID 83525-0136

Publications Referenced Herein:

121 Ways to Live 121 Years,
Dr. Ronald Klatz, MD, DO
Dr. Ronald Goldman PhD, FAASP, DO, FAOASP.
Copyright 2005 by authors, American Academy of Anti-Aging Medicine;
www.worldhealth.net

Nutrition Secrets, Felicia Busch
Copyright 2000, Bottom Line Books,
Boardroom, Inc.
281 Tresser Blvd., Stamford, CT 06901

Power Aging, Gary Null, PhD
Copyright 2003 Gary Null's Anti-aging Center
Bottom Line Books, 281 Tresser Blvd., Stamford, CT 06901

Testosterone for Life, Abraham Morgentaler, M.D.;
Harvard Health Publications, Harvard Medical School; copyright 2011.

Textbook of Bio-Identical Hormones.
Edward D. Lichten, M.D., FACS
Copyright 2007, Edward D. Lichten, Birmingham, MI 48012- 0843

*Understanding Vitamins and Minerals,The Prevention Total Health System
by the Editors of Prevention Magazine;* Copyright 1984, Rodale Press, Inc.
Emmaus, PA 18098-0099

Power Your Life with Positive Thinking, Norman Vincent Peale,
Copyright 1988, Foundation for Christian Living,
P.O. Box FCL, Pawling, NY 12564

Just As I Am: The Autobiography of Billy Graham,
Copyright 1997, Billy Graham Evangelistic Assoc.,
Harper Collins Publishers, New York, NY 10022

For Further Reading:

Living Meaningfully – Practical Help for a Victorious Life, Jim Heckathorn; (Nashville, TN 97222, American Christian Writers Press) 2008, Morningstar Meadow, P.O. Box 136, Elk City, ID 83525

Endnotes

1. Dr. Ronald Klatz, Dr. Ronald Goldman; *121 Ways to Live 121 Years*, (American Academy of Anti- Aging Medicine), p. 129

2. Jerry Menges, *Discover Magazine*; (Charlotte, NC; Billy Graham Evangelistic Association); February 2009; pp. 20,21.

3. Billy Graham, *Just as I am*; (HarperCollins, San Francisco,1997) p 666.

4. Life Extension Magazine, Special Winter Edition 2010 – 2011; p.4

5. Cellular Research Center, St Petersburg, FL 33701

6. Life Extension Foundation, *Disease Prevention and Treatment*, 4th Expanded Edition, Fort Lauderdale, FL, p.705.

7. *Life Extension Magazine*, 2009 Collectors Edition; (Fort Lauderdale, FL); pp. 95-100

8. Dr. Edward D. Lichten; *Textbook of Bio-Identical Hormones*; p.214

9. Lichten,p.213

10. *Life Extension*; pp. 95-100

11. Gary Null, *Power Aging*; (Stamford, CT; Bottom Line Books; 2003); p.62

12. Felicia Busch, *Nutrition Secrets*; (Stamford, CT; Bottom Line Books, Boardroom, Inc.;2000); p.36

13. Julie Ackerman Link, *Above All Love*, (Discovery House Publishers, Grand Rapids, MI 49501, 2008) p.35

14. *Understanding Vitamins and Minerals*; (Emmaus, PA; Rodale Press, Inc, 1984); p.89

15. Life Extension, March 2007, P.62.

16. The Barton Publishing Blog; bartonpublishing.com; 04/15/2011.

17. Roger Mason, The Natural Prostate Cure, Safe Goods, Sheffield, MA 01257; P.27.

18. Roger Mason, ibid, p.40.

19. Lorraine Day, MD, You Can't Improve on God; (Rockford Press, Thousand Palms, CA 92276) video.

20. "Eating Your Way to Prostate Cancer";Life Extension, February2007, pp.33-39

21. Reported in Proceedings of the National Academy of Sciences; September 29, 2003.

22. Dr. David G. Williams, *Alternatives*; (Potomac, MD, Mountain Home Publishing; June 2011); p.1

23. Williams, p.3

24. *Life Extension*, January 2012, pp.38-49

25. The Barton Publishing Blog; www.bartonpublishing.com; 12/11/2010.

26. Life Extension, May 2007, pp.65-67.

27. Ibid, pp. 83-85

28. "An Exercise in Godliness", *Our Daily Bread*; January 2012, (RBC Ministries, Grand Rapids, MI 49501 -2222) Wednesday, January 4, 2012

29. Lloyd J.Ogilvie, *Making Stress Work for You* (Dallas,TX; Word Publishing), pp.181,182

30. *Life Extension*, January 2012, p.30

31. *Dr. Crandall's Heart Health Report*, (Newsmax Media,Inc., West Palm Beach, FL 33409) Vol.2, Issue 3, p.7

32. Ibid, Loraine day, video.

33. William L. Fischer, How to Fight Cancer and Win (Agora Health Books, Baltimore, MD; 2000) pp.160-165.

34. Leslie Taylor, ND *The Healing Power of Rainforest Herbs* (Square One Publishers, Garden City Park, NY 11040, 2005) pp.288-294.

35. Dr. Victor Marchione, Doctors Health Press; (Lombardi Publishing, NY, 10118-0110

36. William Faloon, Misguided Medicine, Life Extension, June 2014, P. 7.

37. Dr. Barbara Starfield, *Journal of the American Medical Association*; Vol.284, No.4, July 26, 2000

38. Starfield

39. Mike Adams, Natural News.Com (online 05/08/2008)

40. Dr. Crandall's Heart Health report, Vol.2, Issue 7, p. 3

41. Kirk Stokel,"Are We all Pre-Diabetic?", Life Extension, Special Winter Edition 2011-2012, p.4

42. Otto Heinrich Warburg, Wikopedia The Free Encyclopedia, online.

43. David G. Williams, MD, http://educate-yourself.org/cancer/benefitsofhydrogen peroxide 17jul03.shtml. July 17, 2003

44. Carl Pradelli, Pain Says Goodbye When You Say Hello, (Nature City, Boca Raton, FL, p. 5.

45. Pradelli, ibid, p.13.

46. Tammy Olsen, *MMS Miracle Book, A Journal of Protocols & Testimonials*;

47. Norman Vincent Peale, *Power Your Life With Positive Thinking*, (Pawling, NY 12564; The Foundation For Christian Living; p.3

48. Peale, p.28

49. Roy L. Smith, *Your Problem is You*, (Nashville, TN; The Upper Room; 1952) p.25